IF JOAN
OF ARC
HAD
CANCER

Johanne

IF JOAN OF ARC HAD CANCER

Finding Courage, Faith, and
Healing from History's Most
Inspirational Woman Warrior

JANET LYNN ROSEMAN, PhD

New World Library
Novato, California

New World Library
14 Pamaron Way
Novato, California 94949

The material in this book is intended for education. It is not meant to take the place of diagnosis and treatment by a qualified medical practitioner or therapist. No guarantee of the effects of using the recommendations can be given nor liability taken.

Unless otherwise indicated, all quotes in this book are excerpts from the trial of Joan of Arc. These excerpts are based on the Orléans manuscript, which is considered the most accurate source, and are taken from the standard English translation of that manuscript, *The Trial of Joan of Arc: Being the Verbatim Report of the Proceedings from the Orleans Manuscript*, trans. W. S. Scott (London: Folio Society, 1956).

Pp. 85–86: Lines from "Anthem" excerpted from *Stranger Music: Selected Poems and Songs* by Leonard Cohen. Copyright © 1993 Leonard Cohen. Reprinted by permission of McClelland & Stewart, a division of Random House of Canada Limited, a Penguin Random House Company.

Text design by Tona Pearce Myers

Library of Congress Cataloging-in-Publication Data
Roseman, Janet Lynn.
If Joan of Arc had cancer : finding courage, faith, and healing from history's most inspirational woman warrior / Janet Lynn Roseman, PhD.
    pages   cm
Includes bibliographical references.
ISBN 978-1-60868-318-5 (paperback) — ISBN 978-1-60868-319-2 (ebook)
1. Cancer—Patients—Life-skills guides. 2. Cancer—Patients—Conduct of life. 3. Cancer—Patients—Attitudes. 4. Joan, of Arc, Saint, 1412–1431 I. Title.
RC262.R65 2015
616.99'4—dc23   2014042453

First printing, March 2015
ISBN 978-1-60868-318-5
Printed in the USA on 100% postconsumer-waste recycled paper

 New World Library is proud to be a Gold Certified Environmentally Responsible Publisher. Publisher certification awarded by Green Press Initiative. www.greenpressinitiative.org

10 9 8 7 6 5 4 3 2 1

For Toby — my eternal guiding light,
whose courage, kindness, and wisdom
I draw from each and every day of my life

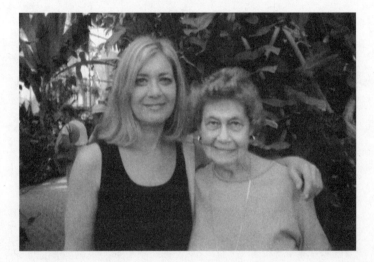

CONTENTS

PART TWO
GATEWAYS TO COURAGE
WITH JOAN OF ARC   115

INTRODUCTION

Welcome to the wisdom of Joan of Arc. This book was written especially for you. Perhaps you are in the process of treatment, healing, or taking care of someone who is seriously ill, and seeking tools of empowerment for yourself or for someone you love. Life is never the same after a diagnosis of cancer, and feelings of vulnerability and anger are understandable and very common. However, the opportunity to change life for the good can also be a part of that truth. Joan of Arc can be your guide as you reclaim your personal wisdom in the shadow of cancer because discovering your personal wisdom is fundamental to your journey.

I believe that the key to this process is the remembering and resurrection of one's personal power in all realms: mind, body, and spirit. These areas are too often overlooked by healthcare professionals who have received little training in the psychological and spiritual aspects of illness. As a result, they are more comfortable focusing on treatment protocols. They fail to realize that this is *not enough* for you, the patient and the human being sitting in front of them. Sacred conversations can occur when you feel safe enough to share the deepest parts of yourself with your physician and other healthcare providers in order to discuss all the dimensions of illness and subsequent healing. When these discussions take place, you and your medical team can create an opening together toward heartfelt connection that can be meaningful for all of you. This book can help you explore your new self and resurrect the powerful woman that you are, who happens to have cancer. Cancer may be your diagnosis, but it is not *your definition*.

As a medical educator and former clinician working with people with cancer using integrative medicine techniques, I truly understand the psychological, spiritual, and physical toll that a cancer diagnosis can extract. Over a decade-long journey with my mother, who had a rare cancer, and my father, who was also diagnosed, I had the privilege of accompanying them as their health advocate through the doors of countless hospitals, doctors' offices, and recovery rooms across the country. In addition, my experiences with clients in healing sessions have taught me a great deal. I have worked with many women, listening to their stories as they shared their cancer journeys with me. I cherish those moments, and I appreciate their willingness to allow me to see inside their world and to learn how their medical experiences transformed their lives.

My wish is that during this life-altering time, you will discover messages from your "truest self," gain insight, and be provided with sustenance and wisdom with Joan of Arc as your companion. This book can help you access your internal courage, activate your own healing process, and honor your unique journey. Admittedly, accessing internal courage during the trauma of diagnosis and treatment is difficult; however, your courage is silently waiting beneath the surface, ready to be unearthed when you are ready.

Why Joan of Arc?

I like to visit consignment stores because I enjoy the exploration and the fact that you can often unearth treasures. A few months after my mother's passing, in an attempt to distract myself from the emotional pain I was feeling, I asked her to send me a "sign" that would indicate that she was with me. Wandering around one of my favorite haunts, I heard a loud thump and looked around to see what had happened. A large painting had fallen over, and I picked it up. The painting was a vintage depiction of Joan of Arc confidently riding her horse with her sword held high. At that moment, I knew this was my mother's sign to me because she knew that I was in need of courage — frightened of living in what had become an unfamiliar world without her — and that resurrecting my courage was terrifying. I spent the next few months immersed in all things Joan and reading everything I could find about her life. The more I read, the more I became convinced that Joan of Arc would be the model for my next book, this book, for she was the ideal inspiration for any woman traversing a difficult passage. After reading the original text of her trial, I was impressed by her humor, bravado, moxie, and never-ending faith in herself.

She is the perfect choice to honor you. Perhaps you have been drawn into or experienced the prevailing cultural belief that "people with cancer are weak," which is not the case at all. My experiences have taught me that people living with cancer (or any other serious illness) possess great courage, enviable courage. This book celebrates that fact. After your diagnosis or during your treatments, you may have received advice from well-meaning but ill-informed people who assert that you are responsible for your illness because of perceived "negative thinking." They may have told you that "if only you would change your point of view," then you would be cancer free. If only life were that simple! Life is a mystery, and unfortunately, we don't have all the answers to the "why" questions. Although everyone is entitled to their belief system, the advice is dismissive, if not dangerous, and victimizes any person with a serious illness. I have also discovered that usually the advice is delivered by people who have never had a personal experience of serious illness. These conversations are very frustrating, and if you examine the lives of the saints who suffered enormous health problems, you realize that they were hardly "negative thinkers" — on the contrary, they were mystics and sages of the highest spiritual order.

Positive thinking, exercise, great nutrition, excellent medical care, personal empowerment, and the provision of emotional and spiritual support can all offer tremendous healing in the midst of any life challenge. However, I also believe that attending to all of your feelings — the dark as well as the light — can be healing as well. All of the emotions — happiness, rage, sadness, anger — have their proper place in the flow of our life; it is when we suppress and judge our emotions and when we dishonor their messages that difficulties arise. You will find exercises in this book to help you identify your feelings, and I urge you to be honest with yourself to derive maximum benefit from these exercises. Self-reflection and self-knowledge provide valuable insights that will help you take charge of your healing journey so you can decide what is best for you.

Creating an "army of support" requires educating your healthcare providers about what you need. The medical culture is wounded; but it is slowly changing, and you can be a primary force for eliciting that change. The role you can play in their humanistic education is invaluable. Don't be afraid to expect more from your care — care that respects all parts of you and includes not only the physical body, but the emotional and spiritual components.

I didn't know that my mother's illness would be the catalyst for my life's work in healing, and she is the inspiration I often draw upon, especially when I am feeling particularly frustrated or vulnerable. This book pays tribute to her and others I have loved and lost. Her courage, much like Joan of Arc's, was palpable.

This book is a guide to help you through the many dimensions of illness and your subsequent healing journey. It is my heartfelt wish that this book will help you summon the inner strength, fortitude, and perseverance you will need and do possess. Although her path was quite formidable, Joan of Arc never gave up on her convictions. Imagine a teenager, a young girl in the fifteenth century without any experience in battle, claiming that *she* would lead France to glory. Her quest seems totally outrageous. She endured ridicule and harassment, and ultimately gave her life, but she never wavered in her belief in herself.

There are many versions of Joan of Arc's trial that you can find online or in books, and it is interesting that many of the statements attributed to Joan differ. Although her words may not be exactly the same in each history book or translation, Joan of Arc's historical contributions are never questioned. I chose to use W. S. Scott's version because I was drawn to the words he inscribed beneath the title: "Being the verbatim report of the proceedings from the Orleans Manuscript." I believe it reflects the actual words that Joan spoke, carefully selected from the transcripts of her trial, held in 1431. During her trial, the proceedings were written down verbatim in French by a notary and his two assistants, who collaborated at the end of each day to produce the text of the transcripts. The original notes were never found, although there is an abbreviated version called the d'Urfé manuscript that is now housed in the Bibliothèque Nationale in Paris. In 1435, the official transcript, known as the Authentic Document (which had been translated from the original French into Latin), was produced by the vice inquisitor from the trial, and four copies were made and sent to the pope, the king, the judge from the trial, and the notary, with the original remaining in the vice inquisitor's possession. All five were sealed and certified as correct. However, historians believe that these transcripts do not contain Joan's exact words and that her testimony was intentionally falsified to prove the claim that she was a heretic. The official report is from the notes of Guillaume Manchon and other notaries by Thomas de Courcelles, but his version was intentionally falsified. A woman successfully leading men into battle and claiming to hear voices from God was unheard-of not only for her time, but for any time. When she refused to alter one word of her narrative during her trial, proclaiming that she only took direction from Divine guidance, it cost Joan of Arc her life. She was a woman well versed in her power and willing to pay the ultimate price for reclaiming it.

The Authentic Document was published in 1902, followed by other editions in 1931 and 1956. The Orléans manuscript, which resides in the Bibliothèque Municipale d'Orléans, is considered the most authentic because it was directly copied from the original French version and reflects Joan's actual statements.

If Joan of Arc Had Cancer is much more than words. It is a book of sacred guidance. Use each section of this book when you are in need of reinforcement, and support that can guide you during your journey. The second section of the book, called Gateways to Courage, will help you explore in depth the themes in the first section. Take your time to explore and work with the Flames of Courage in part 1. I suggest that you read a theme a day (one Flame of Courage every day) for a month. Part 1 contains meditations that can help you access your inner knowing in preparation for the Gateways to Courage in part 2. The Gateways will help you explore in depth the themes from part 1. Each Gateway contains art and guided visualizations that mirror the corresponding themes in the Flames of Courage section of the book. You may wish to work with one theme from the Flame section during one reading session and return on another day, when you have uninterrupted time, to go deeper into that theme by reading the corresponding Gateway. There is no right way to use this book, only *your* way. Feel free to allow Joan of Arc to inspire you by using this book in a manner that feels right for you and addresses your desires and needs.

Everyone needs and deserves support and encouragement in life, but when navigating cancer, often you require more than that. This book will serve and guide you to resurrect the strength, courage, and wisdom that I know you hold. You have the same inner fortitude that Joan possessed. Let her be your companion on your journey, an ally you can count on.

About Joan of Arc

Joan of Arc's achievements are extraordinary for her time, or any time in history, and it is quite tempting to think of her as myth, legend, or folklore. However, Jeanne la Pucelle, or "Joan the Maid," as she liked to be called, was flesh and blood. The daughter of a farmer, this teenager led more than twelve thousand French militia to victory over the English, without any military training or experience riding horses or carrying a sword. Although she restored the rightful place of Charles VII, the dauphin, as king of France, he betrayed her. When she was captured in 1430 and literally sold to the English, who would later sentence her to death, the king did nothing to intervene on her behalf.

This young woman who heard "voices" from God was both a mystic and a visionary. When she was sixteen years old, her father had a prophetic dream that she would ride off to battle. Echoing the limited traditional roles for young women of that era (marriage, celibacy, or prostitution), he believed she would disgrace the family if the dream were fulfilled. How could she possibly ride into battle as the leader and not the courtesan? Because of the dream, he hastily arranged a marriage to keep Joan in line. She was so enraged that she challenged her father in court, disputing the arranged marriage and arguing that she wanted to be a *free* woman. The members of the court were so impressed by her impassioned pleas that they granted her request. This was an exceptional situation in the early 1400s. The theme of the "free woman" would be immortalized over four hundred years later, when Joan of Arc was chosen to be the spiritual icon of the women's suffragette movement, honoring both her courage and her political savvy.

Joan was never taught to read or write and spent her days like most young girls of her time: sewing, tending to her family's farm, and attending church with her mother. Yet she would be transformed from a simple, innocent teen into a mystic and military general. Defying the conventions of her time and cloaked in men's clothing, she became the commander in chief of an army, leading men into battle countless times, although she claimed during her trial that she never killed anyone. Her quest was both a mystical and a spiritual journey, because she devoted her life to God. The fact that she was able to convince royalty, French commanders, and the French people that *she* alone could save France from the assaults of the English and Burgundian troops occupying half of France, and presumed annihilation at their hands, is the stuff of legend. However, Joan made good on her promises.

Tragically, she was used by the king, Charles VII, whose royal reign on the throne he owed to Joan's intelligence in military strategy. When she lost two important military battles, her supporters, believing that these losses indicated that she no longer had the "ear" of God, withdrew their backing and sought a way to get rid of her. When she was captured during a battle at Compiègne, the king seized the moment by doing nothing at all to help her. He was insecure and very unhappy with Joan's ever-increasing fame and adoration, which he believed only he, a royal, was entitled to. Although she still had legions of fans, he used her as his political pawn, knowing that she would be condemned to death; this was the perfect solution for him — her destruction.

She spent eight long months in prison, chained to her bed, even before her famous trial began. The records indicate that Joan slept with two pairs of irons on her legs, attached by a chain very tightly to another chain that was connected to the foot of her bed, itself anchored by a large piece of wood five or six feet long.

Deprived of sleep, food, and emotional support from family and friends, she received her only sustenance from the spiritual balm that was offered to her by her voices and the spiritual visions that guided her each day. It is stunning to realize that during a five-year period, Joan received over 750 messages and visions, communications that she refused to deny. She had her first vision when she was thirteen years old: she heard a voice that "was hardly ever without a light and after she had heard it three times, she knew it was the voice of an angel." She believed this was the voice of Saint Michael, and during her short life, she would also be visited by Saint Catherine and Saint Margaret, whom she described during her trial as wearing beautiful crowns upon their heads.

The court records reflect that during her trial, although the court members (called "inquisitors") tried to break her will, her demeanor grew stronger as she consistently spoke boldly, fiercely, and articulately. They misrepresented her previous testimony to try to confuse her, and it was not unusual for them to show up in her prison cell at all hours of the night, demanding that she answer questions.

During the trial, she did not change her story even when threatened with death. However, in a moment of coercion and misunderstanding, she was forced to sign documents that she believed would earn her release from prison — documents that declared she was a heretic and had lied about her visions. The fact that she wore men's clothing was considered her ultimate disobedient act and was particularly revolting to the men who admonished her during her trial. The documents she signed, called cedulas, or orders of authorization, included the demands that she would only wear women's clothing, never carry arms, and submit to the church's wishes. The second document was of particular significance because it included retractions of everything that she had said during the trial and, more important, a denial of ever hearing voices. It is easy to understand why Joan — who had been chained to her bed for months, assaulted emotionally (and, in the opinion of many scholars, physically), and humiliated and intimidated daily — would agree to sign these documents, especially since she couldn't read a word of any of the papers in front of her.

When she realized what she had done, she proclaimed that she was misled: "I did not say nor did I mean to say that I retracted my apparitions; everything that I have done, I have done out of fear of fire. I have retracted nothing except what was against the truth. I didn't understand what was written on the notification of retraction." But it was too late. On May 30, 1431, Joan of Arc was burned at the stake as a heretic. It is said that her body was reduced to ashes but her heart remained intact, and for her devoted followers, this was further proof of her saintliness and a manifestation of the miraculous.

In 1455, her mother appealed to a papal court at Notre-Dame Cathedral in an effort to restore her daughter's reputation and the defiled family name, arguing with skill that Joan had been deceived: "Certain enemies betrayed her (Joan) in a trial concerning the Faith, and...without any aid given to her innocence in a perfidious, violent and iniquitous trial, without shadow of right...they condemned her in a damnable and criminal fashion and made her die cruelly by fire."

This time, supporters who were prevented from testifying on her behalf at her original trial — including her mother, friends of the family, and soldiers who fought with her in battle — were allowed to speak. After three months of investigations and hearings, her sentence as a "heretic" was declared "null and void." More than four hundred years after her death, Joan of Arc was declared a saint by Pope Benedict XV.

Mark Twain was a huge fan of Joan of Arc. He was so enamored of her and impressed by her significance that he wrote a biography of Joan entitled "Personal Recollections of Joan of Arc" for *Harper's Magazine* in 1896, using the pseudonym Sieur Louis de Conte, her purported page and secretary. The articles later appeared in book form that same year. He wrote, "Joan of Arc, that wonderful child... that spirit which in one regard has had no peer and will have none.... Search as you may, and this cannot be said of any other person whose name appears in profane history." His tribute to her is passionate and typical of his irreverent writing style:

> When we reflect that her century was the brutalist, the wickedest, the rottenest in history since the darkest ages, we are lost in wonder at the miracle.... She was truthful when lying was the common speech of men; she was honest when honesty was become a lost virtue; she was a keeper of promises when the keeping of a promise was expected of no one;... she was steadfast when stability was unknown, and honorable in an age which has forgotten what honor was; she was a rock of convictions in a time when men believed in nothing...; she was unfailingly true in an age that was false to the core; she maintained her personal dignity unimpaired...; she was of dauntless courage when hope and courage had perished.... The work wrought by Joan of Arc may fairly be regarded as ranking any recorded in history, when one considers the conditions under which it was undertaken, and the obstacles in the way.

Joan of Arc lived her flame of courage, and in the next section, you will learn how you can access your own.

Finding Your Flame of Courage

Living with a diagnosis of cancer immediately suggests the expectations of vulnerability — physical, emotional, and spiritual. This perceived vulnerability can actually be an asset, and throughout the twists and turns on the path, you can transmute the meaning of vulnerability from *something less than* into *something more than*. By its very nature, cancer cracks open the portals of life, from "what was" to "what is." During this journey, there are no set rules to follow. You are unique and not only have opportunities to make life-changing choices about treatment, but can rethink the types of emotional and spiritual support you need, discarding what no longer serves.

Each person on this journey has her own perspective and place of attention. The laws of physics dictate that any focus or object of attention requires energy. In this case, I am suggesting that this energy can be attentive to the spiritual and psychological components of healing — components that are fundamental to the cancer journey. The mysteries of the human being are boundless, and from my professional and personal experience, I believe that a diagnosis of cancer or any serious illness can offer the opportunity for travel on the mystical path. This sacred path is highly personal and distinctive. It is a Divine opening for discovery and can happen when one's heart is pierced to the very core. Maximizing one's challenges and tragedies for benefit is the essence of learning for all of us. This education can assist you in accessing an interior wisdom that can elevate your health challenges to become a force for your greater good, and during the process, activate consciousness and guide you to the discovery of the courage inside you. Many people with cancer are keenly aware of this mystical quality and have discovered that cancer also presents a transcendent aspect inside the illness. These opportunities are not confined to a particular stage of cancer, because healing has many faces.

Cancer can be revelatory and contains elements both of destruction and transmutation. The sadness of the body, and the frustration, anger, and rage at even having a cancer diagnosis, are all healthy and genuine responses, especially when one is initially diagnosed or in treatment. Expressing these emotions can be quite healing, and suppressing them undermines the therapeutic process. It is important to find a safe place for this expression, and the exercises offered in part 2, the Gateways, can provide you with that safe forum and give you permission to authentically feel without following the prevalent philosophy that you need to always be strong and fight.

Often when you surrender and give yourself permission to experience and express the full spectrum of emotions — negative, positive, and everything in between — the opportunity for a catharsis is available. It takes a courageous person to be willing to name and explore all of her feelings. However, when you give voice to true feelings, you may discover that the perceived "negative" feelings no longer possess the same power over you. The emotions you have held captive can be heard and consequently can flow through you without getting stuck in your body or psyche.

Joan of Arc knew the importance of expressing her emotions, and throughout her trial, she continued to speak of her visions, convictions, and faith in God. She adhered to her own honorable code even when she was oppressed. Her flame of courage was her strength and commitment to herself even when others were invested in her destruction.

Your flame of courage has a voice that often speaks. It is revelatory and may ask you to reclaim your personal power even when you think it is lost. Cancer requires the fight of an unfamiliar battle (or a returning battle) with a personal sword and shield, and asks you to pay attention to what you may have previously overlooked. It forces us to be attentive to our bodies, our relationships, and our emotional terrain and examine all of the details, to strip us down to the core, which is full of beauty.

The Art of Wabi Sabi

The Japanese have a beautiful word for this consciousness: *wabi sabi*, a concept that allows the discovery of beauty and is considered an art form. The best and most poignant description of wabi sabi that I have found is this: "the simplicity of wabi sabi...as the state of grace arrived at by a sober, modest, and heartfelt intelligence." And the best explanation of how to achieve wabi sabi that I've read advises, "Pare down the essence, but don't remove the poetry."

This invisible connective tissue of all things, wabi sabi strives to recombine all of the elements into a form that has deep meaning. Wabi sabi is often described as the art of imperfection. The triad that forms wabi sabi is simplicity, tranquility, and naturalness. These core aesthetics can easily be a philosophy for women with cancer. Simplicity, by its very nature, implies the paring down of what does and what does not serve, not only in art, but in life. It is the simplicity of choosing what is most useful: physically, spiritually, and emotionally. The act of clearing out what is no longer needed, to form something new, is required. What could you choose? Tranquility provides us with a reassuring curative, and often an accompanying sense of contentment, no matter how our outer life appears. It can also offer a pronounced clarity. Joan's visions and spiritual vows provided her with an invaluable sense of tranquility amid the chaos of her trials. My mother's tranquility lived in the majestic panorama of surrender — surrendering to her feelings. The measure of her courage was often found in her vulnerability and her willingness to express that vulnerability without fear. Naturalness suggests authenticity without artifice. Joan's extraordinary poise, and even sense of humor, during her trial were natural for her. Everyone has their own core of authenticity, though rarely do people reveal that core to the world.

Wabi sabi is the natural transformation and evolution of all things that contain not only "beauty," but imperfection. I believe this beauty resides in the imperfections of who we are, whether we have a cancer diagnosis or not. Wabi sabi celebrates the dents, the rough edges, the scars, the wounds, the blood, the pain of cancer with all its devastation, and allows them to reorganize into something splendid. I fervently believe that these so-called woundings are actually where the beauty resides. Joan of Arc would have embraced this philosophy, for she lived wabi sabi by finding honor in the darkest of places. Can you?

Guidance with Joan of Arc: How to Use This Book

If Joan of Arc Had Cancer is divided into two parts: Flames of Courage and the Gateways. Because your intuitive mind is activated by each Flame of Courage theme, it can be beneficial to work with both sections of this book during the same sitting; however, that is not the only way. The Flames can be read in order for thirty-one days, a new theme each day for one month, or you can choose to work with the sections out of order, depending on your relationship to the themes identified in the book. Always trust your judgment.

Part 1 presents thirty-one Flames of Courage — attributes each based on a particular theme. Each Flame is explained in detail, and many are accompanied by the actual words Joan spoke during her trial, to reinforce the Flame. Following this text is a message from Joan that was intuitively written, and a corresponding meditation and directive. I wrote these messages from Joan of Arc by connecting with her energy during my own meditations. As an experienced intuitive healer, I am comfortable with the practice of "listening" in order to make connection with the spiritual realms.

Part 2 contains thirty-one Gateways to Courage, each corresponding to and expanding on the themes of the Flames of Courage. The Gateways encourage you to cultivate your internal brand of courage and reclaim your personal power using contemplative exercises, narrative, and art. Many of the exercises in this book are based on my experience leading workshops with women with cancer and have proved to be powerful and healing. The Gateways offer you additional opportunities to reach deeper and explore your lived experiences in a safe and sacred arena, to become the heroine of your own journey.

You will notice that the instructions in each section do

not dictate specific responses, and offer open-ended opportunities to evoke and access your internal wisdom. Some of the themes explored suggest concrete ideas, and offer you guidance including "seeking a second opinion" or "creating an army of support," while other sections are devoted to deeper psychological and spiritual study. The methods were designed to help you connect deeply with your authentic self to provide emotional sustenance, especially important for readers who are working with this book without the support of family and friends.

When Do I Use This Book?

If Joan of Arc Had Cancer was written to be used whenever you have the need for guidance, courage, or reflection. You may choose to read a particular Flame of Courage theme before you go to your doctor's appointment (traditional or integrative practitioner), consult with an herbalist or nutritionist, have chemotherapy or radiation treatments, or when you are feeling particularly vulnerable. You can explore the options that work for you. Some women have told me that they have copied the image of Joan of Arc and brought her with them to their treatments and meditated during that time. I encourage you to make this book your own and find *your* way.

Meditation as a Healing Modality

Each Flame of Courage in part 1 provides a suggested meditation for you to follow, and I encourage you to participate.

The healing powers of meditation are well documented and meditation has both a calming and a restorative effect on the body. I have discovered, as I hope you will, that a committed meditation practice opens opportunities for self-knowledge, guidance, self-healing, and engagement with the spiritual realms. You may wish to make an audio recording of each meditation so that you can listen to the instructions without opening and closing the book, and enjoy the process more. If you are working with the book with a friend, you can take turns reading the meditations for each other's benefit.

Feel free to improvise on the suggested meditation in any way that appeals to you. You may find that, over time, you'll wish to add further elements to a particular meditation, such as free writing, drawing, or painting — all elements you can preserve in the pages of a journal. Use the meditations in this book to your greatest advantage to discover what is best for you and what makes sense for you.

There are countless ways to meditate besides formal practices, and you may wish to experiment and expand your beliefs. I believe that drawing, writing, gardening, cooking, coloring, or even walking can be forms of meditation. In my life, ballet has served as my healing meditation because the physical movement and visceral attention needed during ballet class help me to move my attention from mind into body.

The common thread of any type of meditation practice (whether it is active or passive) is "presence." You are present in the moment and not thinking about yesterday, tomorrow, or next week — you are simply present to yourself. This is really the beauty of any meditation because it allows you to be truly available to forge connections with spiritual, some might say Divine, principles.

The Process of Meditation

Take a moment to acquaint yourself with how to meditate, using the meditation exercise below. (As previously noted, it can be helpful to make an audio recording of the meditations in this book, including the one that follows, so you'll have the freedom to go deep without consulting the book's pages, able to participate fully in the process.) Choose a time when you know you will not be interrupted, and if necessary, take the phone off the hook, turn off your cell phone, and even put a sign on the door that declares, "Do not disturb!" Make sure you are wearing comfortable clothing and take off your shoes. You can meditate while sitting or lying down; the choice is yours. If you are sitting in a chair, uncross your legs and let your hands rest gently on your knees or by your side.

> **MEDITATION.** Close your eyes and imagine a blank movie screen in front of you. Allow your mind to witness the day's events — and all that you are thinking about. When you are ready, mentally project these thoughts onto this blank screen; and fill it with all your concerns. Breathe. This movie screen is large enough to hold all your worries in this moment. You may notice that as you release your thoughts, it is easier to concentrate on your breath. Breathe deeper. Relax your jaw, your face, and any areas of your body that may be holding tension. Put your hands on your belly and feel the breath as it

enters your body; and notice the lightness of your breath as you exhale.

Continue to breathe and notice how the screen in front of you that was filled with thoughts and worry is slowly turning blank. Enjoy this quiet and let your breath fill you with energy and a feeling of lightness and calm. Keep breathing and know that the information you will receive during your meditations will always be for your best and highest good. Notice any tension in your body and allow yourself to be liberated from thoughts. You do not have to think about anything; you do not have to do anything; just be present in this moment. Continue to breathe as you notice you are feeling more relaxed and comfortable. If you fall asleep, that is fine. This meditation is for you. Remind yourself that you are able to feel this deep relaxation and calm whenever you wish. Keep breathing.

Imagine that there are large anchors at the bottom of your feet. The anchors can be made of any materials that you wish. Imagine sending these anchors down deep into the floor (below your carpet — if you have one), below the foundation of your home. Send them below your home, into the firm ground. These anchors will hold you and allow you to firmly inhabit your body during your meditation. Once the anchors are deeply embedded in the earth, continue to breathe, knowing you are safe, you are protected, and you are at peace. Whenever you are ready (and there is no time limit), gently open your eyes. You will probably feel a renewed sense of calm and peace, and perhaps a tingling sensation as the energies of your body are circulating.

GROUNDING

When you return to the outer world after a meditation, it is important that you ground yourself. I enjoy the anchoring meditation shown above, because it places me firmly in my body and allows me to feel "held" by the earth. Some people who are not used to meditating can feel a little dizzy afterward. So, after meditating, it is always good to take the time to shake out your hands and feet, and slowly stand up, to return to ordinary consciousness. Stamp the floor so that you can truly reinhabit your body completely. It is also helpful to drink a glass of water to rehydrate yourself.

If you are unfamiliar with the meditation process, I suggest that you take a week or so to practice and experience meditating before using this book.

The Intuitive Process

If you wish to go through this book sequentially, beginning with the first Flame of Courage, moving on to the second Flame, and so on, please do so; however, you can also work with this book using intuitive techniques. The intuitive process is a wonderful practice that can help you build your confidence to the point that you truly trust and believe that you have the innate wisdom to identify the theme that is most important for you to explore at this moment. We all possess intuitive abilities, and for some, these abilities are more familiar and easier to access, because of practice and experience. This book will help you enhance your intuitive abilities. If you would like to explore how to work with your intuition, try the following exercise.

> Put your hand on the headings in this book's table of contents and close your eyes. When you feel connected to a particular theme, place your finger on that heading, or you can place your finger where you feel drawn. You can flip through those pages in the book and decide if that is where you want to begin reading. You may be surprised to discover that your selection is a topic you are attracted to at this time in your life and need to investigate further at this point in your journey. This is a process of intuitive wisdom.

Working with Intention

There is another way to use this book that you may find helpful. This is the "way of intention" that calls forth your innate wisdom and purpose. By working with intention, you can amplify the synergy of your thoughts with Joan's wisdom. Intention allows you to direct your thoughts with clarity and focus. When you declare to yourself that "you will be well," this is intention. Think about this sacred intention as a vibrant, precise ray of white light that you can access whenever you like. Joan of Arc used her power of intention throughout her life and trusted her inner knowing at all times. She knew that she was being led by Divine guidance, although her voices did not always reveal the complete plan to her — just the information she needed at the time. Trust that you will receive information that will help you each time you use this book. The following exercise can guide you to working with the way of intention.

> Think about what wisdom you wish to know at this time in your life and create it in the form of a question. Write it down. Once you have formulated your question (working with one question at a time), concentrate on that thought deeply to focus it like a beam of light. The following options will help you locate the theme to explore during this session:
>
> - Open part 1 of the book at random to receive the information that addresses your question.
> - Look through the table of contents and locate the theme toward which you feel the strongest intuitive pull.
> - Open the book to the table of contents, close your eyes, and while keeping your question in mind, choose a theme by using your finger like healing radar to guide you to the proper heading to work with.
> - Write down all the headings listed in the table of contents on slips of colored paper and place them in a bowl, and with your question in mind, close your eyes and select a slip of paper that will intuitively identify the proper theme to work with to address your needs.
>
> Once you have identified the theme you need to work with, take a few breaths and close your eyes,

trusting that the information you receive will be the exact wisdom from Joan of Arc that you need. Make notes in the journal that you have dedicated to the exploration of the sections in this book, to chronicle your relationship with Joan. Many women find it helpful to place her picture in their office, bedroom, or other "room of their own" to amplify her presence.

Aligning with Joan of Arc

Before you begin reading, complete the following writing exercise, which is designed to help you connect with Joan's legacy of courage and strength. Please allow her to guide you.

You will be writing for this exercise, so you will need paper or a favorite notebook. You will be answering a short list of questions using the "freewriting" method. This method asks you to write down whatever comes to mind, truthfully, without editing or thinking about the "correct" response, and without trying to make the writing perfect. Let your pen guide you. There is great wisdom in this method, and it was not chosen haphazardly. In my experience teaching writing/healing workshops, I have discovered that when you give yourself permission to write down your responses without using the logical mind, you can circumvent thought and begin to access your intuitive voice. This intuitive voice was the foundation of Joan's life — a voice she trusted wholeheartedly.

Answer the following questions and write whatever thoughts arrive using the freewriting method, and without censoring yourself.

- What do you hope to learn from this book?
- What particular wisdom would you like to access from Joan of Arc to help you on your medical journey today?
- What does Joan of Arc mean to you symbolically or spiritually?

Take some time to reflect on what you wrote and examine whether any particular theme comes alive, perhaps one that you may not have given thought to before. You may be surprised by what you wrote or discover that feelings you may not have allowed yourself to possess are now consciously surfacing. Please be aware that there are no right or wrong answers — whatever you wrote is true for *you*. Always trust your writing.

Writing a Statement of Healing

Before you begin working with this book, I would like you to create a Statement of Healing. This statement is an act of commemoration of your courage (even if you don't feel courageous right now) and will help invite Joan's wisdom into your life. Choose a statement that is authentic and speaks to you now, wherever you may be on your cancer journey. The first thought that enters your mind is usually best. Write down all statements that immediately come to you — that have resonance. If you are have difficulties getting started, a universal Statement of Healing you can borrow until your own arrives is "I know I will discover the highest and best healing wisdom for myself at this time in my life."

Some women have told me that before they begin reading, they perform a ritual of sacred invocation that holds special meaning for them. Prayer or sacred invocation of any kind is very powerful, and I encourage you to create your own meaningful rituals while using this book. You may wish to light candles or say a particular prayer when you work with Joan of Arc. It is best to honor your commitment to yourself and your healing by choosing a regular time to use this book each day. You may also prefer to work with Joan only during your treatment sessions or when recovering from procedures or surgeries. Welcome to Joan of Arc's wisdom.

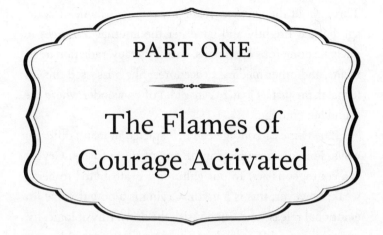

PART ONE

The Flames of Courage Activated

The concept of the flame of courage has a noble history. The military continues to offer the Flame of Courage Award to military personnel for their courageous acts in combat. The metaphor of this flame was not lost on the sculptor Rodin, an artist and astute philosopher who believed that beauty could be retrieved from the flame of one's inner life. Joan of Arc claimed this flame of courage. So can you.

My mother taught me the definition of the flame of courage, especially during the last years of her life. This is not to suggest that she never was angry, frustrated, depressed, or full of rage, because sometimes she was, and so was I. She had a lot to be angry about: Her trusted physician dismissed her cries for help and ignored test results that raised suspicions of cancer. She was never told about that report, and her complaints were not addressed until she sought a second opinion. By that time, her cancer had progressed.

Throughout the next ten years, my mother's flame of courage burned brightly and gave her the internal resources to navigate numerous operations, chemotherapy, radiation treatments, and other medical procedures. She possessed this internal flame just as Joan of Arc did. I often wonder where she found her courage.

The flame of courage can be depicted in many different ways. For some, crying can be one of those forms. Crying is a courageous act. In our culture, it is attributed to being weak; however, this is a myth. Crying is a potent valve for emotional release and can nourish the body. Physiologically, our tears have different chemical components depending on the crying impulse. The tears we shed when we peel onions are not the same tears we shed when we are feeling sad. Our psyche has its own computer that literally punches in the correct physiology of tears to release for different occasions. Crying is a profound act of emotional surrender; and akin to the creation of art, it is a mysterious and private experience. Our tears summon us to pay attention to our bodies and our feelings, but we do not always listen to the call. Our tears pulse with meaning. They are valuable to us, and within the core of our tears rest their sanctity and recuperative power.

Your flame of courage may also be a shield from the world when it is time for reflection and retreat, providing an important psychological barrier of protection. We all possess the ability to create flames of courage, but the blueprint will vary according to the person. Excavating internal strength, surrendering to what is, or the release of tears can all be your flame of courage.

You will find on the following pages the themes of the

Flames of Courage, and I encourage you to take your time to explore them. These Flames of Courage mirror the attributes that Joan of Arc possessed and offer you the opportunity to discover, uncover, and find guidance. It is also an opportunity for you to create sacred space, sacred space that is for you alone. You may want to work alone, or you may decide to share your experiences using the Flames of Courage themes with other women who are also traveling this journey. Remember that these Flames reflect all that Joan of Arc was, and that you can depend on her to guide you during your journey. She is a formidable and kind companion.

‹–⏤◦◉◦⏤–›

VALOR

Among the definitions of valor are "boldness," "determination in facing great danger (especially in battle)," and "heroic courage." *Valor* is derived from the Latin word *valere*, meaning "to be of worth" or "to be strong." The definitions of both *valor* and its Latin root are personified in the life of Joan of Arc. Her remarkable courage is well documented in books and films, and resides in the words she spoke on her own behalf during her trial. She succeeded in crowning a king, defeating the English troops in battle, and lifting the spirits of her people when all hope was lost. You are being reminded today that Joan's valor is available to you. No matter what is happening during your cancer journey, you are being told directly that you too can call upon your own internal "remarkable courage" that you may have forgotten but that dwells inside you. You only have to resurrect that memory.

TRIAL

One of Joan's prized possessions was the sword that she carried with her into battle. The story of how she received that sword is just as magical as her military abilities. She was literally led by her Divine voices to the discovery of the sword — a sword that no one knew existed — inside the Church of

Sainte-Catherine-de-Fierbois. The sword had added meaning for her because Saint Catherine was one of her trusted voices. She told Charles VII, the future king of France, that it would be found lying by the altar. He sent for it, and the sword was found in the exact spot where she claimed it would be. The rusted sword with five crosses engraved on it was given to her, as a gift, for her first battle at Orléans. This was the first time Joan had even seen a sword, much less used one. No doubt the churchmen who discovered the sword were just as startled to find the rusty weapon as she was to receive it.

JOAN SAID

"It was not very deeply buried underground, behind the altar. Just after the sword was found the men of the church gave it a good rubbing and thereupon the rust fell off without effort."

MESSAGE

Remind yourself of a situation in your life when you exhibited valor. It doesn't make a difference if this happened last week or many, many years ago. Make a list of the times when you felt full of valor. Ask yourself the following questions:

Who were the characters in your drama?
How did your body feel when it was full of valor?
How did you feel emotionally?
How long has it been since you felt like this?

Write down the small steps you can take to honor, preserve, and revive those moments of valor in your life now.

Dust off your memory and let the rust fall off so you can use that wisdom now.

MEDITATION

Close your eyes. Think about the word *valor*. Let any images that occur to you arise, and simply watch them appear before you in your mind's eye. Direct your intention clearly and affirm that you wish to receive your truth about the word *valor* from Joan of Arc, a message that speaks to your own life at this time. You may see a symbol or image, or receive words or a message. Document everything you saw or experienced in the pages of your journal so that you will have an important and revelatory record for further reflection.

Flame of Courage 2

PATIENCE

There is a prevailing belief that "patience is a virtue" and that if you don't possess this quality, somehow you are misbehaving. But *patience is not always a virtue*. Unless you have experienced what it is like to wait, you can't really understand the depths of frustration it can cause. Spending hours in the waiting room for a doctor's appointment (or a meeting with a healthcare professional), waiting for the results of medical tests and procedures, or waiting for a report that will shed light on your medical challenges and subsequent treatments *will* test anyone's patience. You know the difficulties. But do you really need to be patient?

Scrutinize your situation. Try to understand if your impatience is truly serving you. Is your impatience justified? This is key. Ask yourself the following questions to find out whether your impatience is a hindrance or a benefit:

> Could there be any complications you aren't aware
>   of (records sent out of state, a second review of
>   tests, physicians out of town)?
> What is a reasonable time frame?
> How long have you been waiting for a return call?

If you are waiting for your appointment in the aptly called "waiting room," you have the right to ask how late your healthcare provider is running that day and whether you can return at another time. If it has been more than a half hour, don't hesitate to ask when you can expect to see your provider.

Don't be afraid to ask questions. Realize that *your time is valuable* and that you cannot be expected to wait for hours on end without any information. Patience takes practice, but be clear whether you are feeling virtuous or your patience is making you a victim.

TRIAL

Joan ventured through enemy territory on horseback for 375 miles from the town of Vaucouleurs to Chinon, where the future deposed king, Charles, lived in exile. He was a "king" the French people had little faith in; Joan was the only person who believed in his destiny, a destiny the messages from her voices had revealed to her. Charles was twenty-six years old, emotionally unstable, and struggling with his mother's claim that he was illegitimate. Just as Joan was about to meet with the dauphin (as she called him), the first of many cross-examinations began. Theologians who were part of his entourage asked her to produce a "sign" from God. Joan was not only fatigued by her long journey; she was also frustrated by the lack of faith the supporters of King Charles showed in her claims.

JOAN SAID

"By the name of God, I haven't come to give signs. Lead me and I will show you the sign for which I have come."

MESSAGE

Sometimes you need to assert yourself and claim your answers! Don't back down or let other people intimidate you. Search for the specific information that will help you in your medical journey. Ask questions and demand answers. Time is of the utmost importance, and I truly understand that struggle. I want you to take control as much as you possibly can, as I did.

MEDITATION

Close your eyes. Take a few moments to think about what the word *patience* means to you. Notice how similar it is to the word *patient*. What images, symbols, memories occur to you? Write them down or draw the images.

When you feel this exercise is complete, take some time to examine the material that has come forward in the meditation and allow this information to reveal any insights.

Flame of Courage 3

SURRENDER

The wide array of sometimes forbidden emotions that arrive and depart and return again can create emotional chaos that is not helpful to you. Second-guessing yourself, self-blame, or playing the "What if?" game has no value to you and is simply destructive. Period. You are being reminded that the more you can allow yourself to surrender and remove these wounding patterns, the more opportunity you have to invite peace of mind into your life. Give yourself permission to surrender your self-doubts completely.

TRIAL

For six days in 1430, Joan learned from her voices that she would be taken prisoner. "My voices told me that I would be captured, that it had to be so, that I should not be amazed but that I should take it favorably."

MESSAGE

Surrender is not an act of self-defeat, and it can be an act of peace — emotional peace — for yourself. Although you may be enveloped by fearful thoughts, you can use your own will to choose to surrender to the "what is" at this moment in your life. Surrender, my dear friend, knowing that you can resurrect yourself emotionally and physically when you are feeling stronger. The act of surrendering can be very empowering and can also provide you with greater insight. How would it feel if you surrendered all of it? Can you relinquish your doubts to trust your healing process?

MEDITATION

Close your eyes and think about what surrender means to you. Does it have a particular texture? A color? A shape or size? Is it located within your body? In what area do you find it? Can you pay attention to its message? Ask yourself if you are ready to surrender to what is occurring in your life.

When you have received your personal message of surrender, you will create a words-of-power statement. A words-of-power statement is akin to an affirmation. It is a series of words, or a single word, that has particular meaning and personal power for your life at this time. Below you will find some words-of-power statements written by other women.

"I surrender my challenges, knowing that I will be safe and protected at all times."

"Although I am terrified of what will happen next, I surrender to my higher wisdom."

"Surrender offers me the opportunity to accept my challenges and to live my life as I see fit."

Feel free to adopt any of these statements until you create your own words-of-power statement.

Flame of Courage 4

⊸⊶⊷◉⊷⊶⊶

PRAYER

Choose a form of prayer for your healing. Prayer is a deeply personal choice, and it is important to honor your personal beliefs about prayer. For some women, traditional prayers from their respective religions are powerful; for others, spiritual prayers do not have a religious connection. The invocation of prayer can be practiced in various locations — a traditional religious setting (such as a church, temple, or mosque), a beautiful garden, a mountaintop, or the privacy of your own bedroom. Painting, dancing, walking — these activities are also prayers if you intend them to be. You may choose to recite prayers from sacred texts or from literary texts you love. You can also create your own prayers, using words that have a particular resonance for you, perhaps the name of a loved one whose heart you hold. The form of prayer you choose must speak to you authentically if it is going to have any personal value. Schedule your prayer ritual during a time of day or night when you are sure you won't be disturbed. Write it down so it becomes an important part of your daily schedule.

TRIAL

When Joan was asked during her trial what words she used when she prayed, she answered, "I beg Our Lord and Our Lady to send me counsel and help and they send it to me."

MESSAGE

Whenever I was confused or scared, I invoked the power of prayer to help me. I didn't know how to lead a military battle or command an army of men. I was terrified. I didn't know what words to speak at my trial, and I prayed so I could hear my voices and listen to their advice. I needed to receive the comfort of their words. I was only a young girl, and I knew that I needed Divine guidance. I could not have accomplished any of these feats without this guidance. You can access Divine guidance for help. Guidance was always provided to me, even when I felt emotionally drained. It will be provided to you as well. I invite you to choose a prayer ritual that you can commit to each day as I did.

MEDITATION

When you think about the word *prayer*, what images come to mind? You may recall your childhood place of worship or a place that currently holds sacred meaning for you. If you aren't feeling well enough to travel to a particular location, that is fine; you don't need to go to a particular setting for sacred guidance. Joan received her visions while she was in prison, hardly a setting that you would imagine offering spiritual direction. She received guidance everywhere — in prison, on the battlefield, and at the end of her life — and so can you. Know that in your meditation, you can create your own sanctuary of prayerful healing, and remember that you can return to this interior place of solace whenever you wish.

Flame of Courage 5

⋄⋅⟶◉⟵⋅⋄

QUIET YOUR MIND

The healing attributes of meditation are well established, and it is no wonder that meditation has been an integral part of the world's spiritual practices. The purpose of meditation is to allow yourself to quiet your mind's frantic thoughts so that you can access a higher wisdom, a wisdom that you possess. Dedicate ten to twenty minutes each day to a meditation practice. Grant yourself the opportunity to become still, clear your mind, and breathe. Pay attention to each breath and release all thoughts of the day. With practice, you will find yourself calmer and better equipped to handle each day's challenges.

TRIAL

During Joan's eight-month prison sentence, she was shackled to her bed at night and forced to wear leg irons during the day. It is extraordinary that, in such extreme circumstances, she had the emotional fortitude to make spiritual contact with the voices she trusted so much. But she did. During her hundreds of spiritual encounters, she received the guidance she needed. It is reassuring that even Joan of Arc admitted she did not know what the next step in her life would be, and she accepted that. She used her prayer meditations to help her through her battles, both on the military fields and while she was imprisoned by English soldiers. Remarkably, through her meditations, she always found a way to create the sacred space she needed, and you can create that same sacred space.

MESSAGE

I was often surrounded by the peculiarities and ugliness of war. I always made time to pray, to meditate, to make contact with my voices. It was this inner world that provided me the strength and courage to go on, even when I often didn't know how. I could not connect with the voices until I was still and quiet, and this form of meditation offered me great peace and comfort, especially when I was alone and scared. Practice quieting your mind so that you can have the tools to calm yourself and remove the fears that may be troubling you, to let the healing powers of the spiritual worlds enfold you.

MEDITATION

Close your eyes. Envision a ray of green light entering your body from the top of your head and let this gentle stream of light travel throughout your entire body. Allow the light to focus on the areas of your body that need special healing. Let this light linger and wrap around the areas that need the most attention. Take all the time you need.

When you are ready, let the green light pass through your body until it reaches the tips of your toes. When you are finished with this light meditation, invite (through your imagination) a vibrant stream of golden light to radiate around you. Let it enfold your body tightly like a well-worn and cozy blanket. You may feel tingling sensations in your body and a deeper sense of calm. Remind yourself that this beautiful blanket of golden light is available to you at all times.

Flame of Courage 6

‹———◇———›

TRUST

Trust your instincts. It is tempting to relinquish your self-trust when you are on a journey that is unfamiliar. Your medical journey is unknown and new terrain for you to travel; however, remember you have also had experiences in your life that were unknown and times when you didn't know where you were headed, but you arrived safely. If you choose to navigate this journey with trust — complete trust in yourself — you have the chance to slowly and effortlessly build a strong, unwavering foundation of emotional independence so that you can regain control during your life's challenges. Know that your instincts are intuitively based and can be trusted now and in the future. The more you live this feeling of trust, the easier it will be to rely on its wisdom. You will make the correct decisions. Trust that your journey can lead you through the process of deep self-discovery.

TRIAL

Joan's mission to save France was one she believed in with all her heart. Her "calling" is best described by a Dominican monk who testified during Joan's nullification trial, which cleared her name as a heretic: "When she was watching over the animals, a voice revealed itself to her, which said that God had great pity on the people of France, and that she had to go into France [from her home on the frontier]. Upon hearing that message, she began to weep, and then the voice bade her to go to [the city of Vaucouleurs], where she would find a captain who would bring her to safety in France unto the king and that she should have no uncertainty. And so she did go to the king's court without delay."

MESSAGE

If you chose to read this Flame of Courage today, I want you to truly know that, yes, your instincts are correct. The inner feelings you have about what is best for your life, whether they are related to your medical decisions or your life's choices, are to be trusted. Pay attention to any intuitive wisdom you are receiving through your feelings, dreams, and, most of all, your inner knowing. I did. Trust yourself even when others do not.

MEDITATION

Close your eyes and envision the word *Trust* emblazoned on a neon sign in front of you. What color is the writing? How large or small is it? Do you recognize the writing style? Hold this image as long as you can. When you are scared, feeling alone or abandoned, recall your neon sign and set it in front of you in your mind's eye. You may also wish to draw it and carry it with you, or post it in a place where you can see it each day, to remind you that you can trust yourself during your healing process.

STRENGTH

Emotional strength is often the catalyst for creating physical strength. The mind can indeed work many wonders. Frequently, athletes in training visualize their goal — they "see" themselves winning a race while embodying and sensing the feeling of victory throughout their body. You can create the emotional strength and inner stamina that you need by knowing there is a never-ending supply that you can draw upon to serve, not sabotage, you. You are being asked to examine carefully your beliefs about just how strong you are.

Look through old photograph albums to find an image of yourself that reminds you of your best self, of a time when you had a strong sense of yourself and your mission in life. Place this image in your bathroom or bedroom so you can receive its power. You are the strong woman in the photograph, and your life continues to have purpose. Select pictures from your favorite magazines that reinforce this attribute, or cut out words that you find inspiring. Create symbols that are meaningful to you, and blend your pictures with other found items to represent the strength you possess.

TRIAL

Joan dictated a letter (since she could not read or write) to the inhabitants of a French village who were waiting for her army to free them, which said: "Joan the Maid sends you her news and begs and demands that you entertain no thoughts about the just quarrel she is pursuing on behalf of the Blood Royal and the French kingdom. I promise and assure you that I will never abandon you as long as I live."

MESSAGE

Call upon me. I am here to guide you. It is not necessary to display physical prowess; let me remind you that you have the necessary inner strength to go forward in your life. Request my help by calling my name and ask that I sit beside you to share my strength with you until you discover your own. I am honored to help you, and I promise and assure you that I will never abandon you.

MEDITATION

Close your eyes and try to clear out all of your mind's ramblings and any thoughts you may have. When you feel relaxed, think about what the word *Strength* means to you and allow a symbol, color, picture, or word come to you. You may also see a particular person from your life (past or present), and if so, know that they are offering their support to you at this time. Just allow the images to come through, and resist the temptation to force a particular symbol or word or image; let it arrive of its own accord. When you are finished, draw any images you received and document any additional information you would like to include.

Flame of Courage 8

HUMOR

Humor is a deflector of negativity. Laughter, like tears, is always healing. You are being asked to bring humor into your life. First, identify what makes you laugh: Do you enjoy children's movies? Iconic comedy shows like *I Love Lucy* or *Seinfeld*? Mel Brooks or Jim Carrey movies? Make the time to watch movies or television programs that can remind you just how terrific it is to laugh. If you have a favorite comedian, take them along with you on a CD and listen to them while you are driving to work or doing your errands. Allow the beautiful gift of laughter to enter your life.

My friend Jane had the most beautiful spirit, and when we were together, she could make me laugh until I cried. Not only was she smart and talented, but we giggled like small children; and I have never met anyone else who could bring out that aspect of my personality.

Take some time and make a list of all the people in your life who have the ability to make you laugh. Look at your list and make some calls to renew your connection with them. Tell them that laughter is your prescription and invite them to be an integral member of your healing team. Ask them to visit or plan a schedule of phone calls so you can rekindle the art of laughter with their support.

TRIAL

The patron saint of France, Saint Michael, was one of the many saints who visited Joan during her visions. In a clumsy attempt to discredit and humiliate her, Joan was asked by her inquisitors if he appeared to her naked. She was probably both irritated and amused by the question and responded with a brash reply: "Do you think that Our Lord does not have the wherewithal to clothe him?"

MESSAGE

You can find humor even in the most serious of situations. I knew that they were trying to humiliate me throughout my trial, particularly whenever they asked me about my visions. Of course, Saint Michael was beautifully clothed when he appeared to me, but I was determined not to give them the satisfaction of answering their interrogations in detail. My visions were private. Find something to laugh about in your life, even with all its current gorges and steep places. My friend, I know that you have the wherewithal to do that.

MEDITATION

Close your eyes and imagine yourself hearing the laughter of someone you love or loved. Listen closely and hear their infectious laugh. Let their laughter get louder and louder, and allow the image of that person to appear before you. Hold this image until you find yourself smiling — even laughing with them again.

COURAGE

Your illness is requiring you to have courage — courage to face your diagnosis head-on; courage to change your life; and courage to continue to create a beautiful life no matter how your life may look right now, simply because you are deserving. Reach deep to locate that courage and take a courageous stance, perhaps the most courageous stance you've ever taken. You are brave. You are gallant. Hold the energies of Joan of Arc within you. Believe that you can find secure footing again and allow your courage to lead you to solid ground.

TRIAL

When Joan of Arc led her devoted militia in combat during the battle of Orléans, she told them to "have no fear," and they believed her. She inspired her troops to fight with honor and bravery during every battle she led. Her command was so intimidating to the enemy that after she won the battle of Orléans, it was not unusual for the opposing forces to retreat when they saw her army approaching.

MESSAGE

I was only a young girl dressed in men's clothing, carrying my sword. I didn't have any military experience at all, but I did have the Divine guiding me. I couldn't even ride a horse! When I first heard the voices, I told them, "I am just a poor girl and know nothing of fighting." I discovered I was on a sacred mission to heal France, just as you are on your own sacred healing mission. Your mission, your only mission right now, is to have courage. If I uncovered my own courage, then so can you. Follow me! Allow me to share my courage with you. I have enough to share with you.

We can get through this next fight together. Let me come to your aid!

MEDITATION

Close your eyes and imagine yourself as a warrior. Take some time to study the way you look. How are you dressed? How are you holding your body? Take your time and examine your image from head to toe. Try to envision inside yourself how it feels to be strong, to be brave, to be ready for anything. What battle are you facing? What type of armor are you wearing? What are you carrying for protection? Do you think the armor you are visualizing is adequate? If not, adjust the image until it feels just right externally and internally. When you are ready, take a moment to meditate on the armor you are wearing and carrying, and think about how you can use that image of protection during your life's current challenges.

Flame of Courage 10

⤙══◎══⤚

COMMEMORATION

Take stock of who you are. It is time to celebrate and commemorate yourself. Examine your accomplishments, no matter how small they may appear to you. Resist the all too familiar temptation to negate your successes. Although there is not a material measure of your strength, bravery, or focused will to heal, all your successes are significant, even the ones you may discount. Write down your achievements so you can recognize the inspiring, beautiful, and amazingly brave person you are. Retrieve this list when you are feeling upset and despairing. Read it *aloud* whenever you need to be uplifted.

TRIAL

Every victory that Joan was able to achieve established her celebrity. She was adored and gained notoriety as a woman of superhuman status; and given her achievements, it is easy to understand why she would be seen as more than a mere mortal. Her remarkable abilities extended to the belief by many that her touch held extraordinary healing powers and people flocked to her — to see her, touch her, and to be enveloped by her Divine energies.

After her victory at Orléans, Joan rode proudly into the

town to celebrate her victory. A woman from the town came forward and asked her to touch her infant, believing that contact with Joan ensured that Joan's extraordinary powers would be transferred directly to her child. Aware of the power of love that is conveyed from mother to child, Joan told her, "Touch her yourself. Your touch is much better than mine!"

MESSAGE

Commemorate yourself! Remember your value! Your deeds, your wisdom, your love, and passions have guided you in the past. Let the remembrance of those successes take you into your future with great pride. Create a ritual of commemoration just for *you*! I am reminding you to take pride in and celebrate your accomplishments.

MEDITATION

Close your eyes. Focus on an achievement that you have had in your life that has particular significance for you. It doesn't matter what the achievement was or what age you were when it occurred. When you have a deep remembering of this time in your life, hold on to this image. Recall how old you were and how you felt at that moment. Reimagine the other participants who shared in your glory and remember how proud you felt. Try to connect with this inner feeling as authentically as possible. Call upon this commemoration whenever you need it. It is a potent prescriptive healing.

Flame of Courage 11

WOUNDING

Wounds contain wisdom and possess great power, particularly when you allow your wounding to be felt and acknowledged. They can be your greatest source of strength and teach you the gift of self-compassion. When you have experienced suffering that splits you open, you have the opportunity to understand the true meaning of the heart of compassion for yourself and for others in your life. Remember that the shattering you are experiencing is part of a transformative process. Trust that you will indeed emerge anew to create beauty from destruction. This is the heroine's journey. Seek the wisdom; seek the message; seek the bold and evolving knowledge that you can find through your wounds.

There are several types of wounding: physical, emotional, and spiritual. You may be experiencing one or more types of wounding. If you can identify that wounding, you can use it to empower yourself. Take a moment and ask yourself whether your wounding is physical, emotional, or spiritual. What type of wounding is being presented to you at this time to help you gain greater self-knowledge? Are you ready to hear its message? How can you attend to your wounding and transmute it into further insight?

TRIAL

During one of her battles, Joan was struck in the neck by an arrow, a wound that her voices told her she would suffer. Her men carried her off the battlefield, trying to shield her from the violent combat zone, and instead of agreeing to be taken to safety in a nearby village, she removed the arrow from her neck and returned to the battle, a battle that she and her men won.

MESSAGE

Nothing can prepare you for facing your wounds because they will be unfamiliar. Even though I was told that I would be injured, I didn't know, truly know, how I would react until it happened. I was astonished by my own strength and ability to summon the inner courage to continue. If you are feeling injured in mind, body, or spirit, attend to these wounds and don't ignore them. Acknowledge them. If it is a physical wound, find appropriate paths to alleviate the pain and seek out help from trusted healers. Emotional and spiritual wounds are usually much deeper; however, the fact that they are invisible does not reduce their impact. Find the emotional and spiritual sustenance and support that you need, from family, friends, and professionals that you feel safe with and can trust. You do not have to go through this alone. I had help from my army of support, and so can you.

MEDITATION

Close your eyes. Think about a wounding experience you have identified. Go deeper and imagine that this wounding has an important message to offer you. Listen. You do not have to reinjure yourself; but listen to the message as an interested observer. Quiet yourself, free yourself from all distractions, and truly listen in the silence. Expect that you will receive wisdom to help you understand your wounding and realize it is your friend and a valuable ally. If you do not receive any direct message immediately, that is fine; there is no time limit. Dream work can be a rich source and a powerful method for activating messages about what you need for your healing process. Before you go to sleep tonight, tell yourself that the inner knowing you seek will be revealed to you through your dreams and that you will remember the communication.

Flame of Courage 12

✦━━◉◎◉━━✦

DIVINE GUIDES

Seek out guidance from a Divine source. When our lives are not working, when we are in extreme emotional, physical, or spiritual pain, we frequently seek out connection to a Divine source. Divine guidance is all around you, ready to be revealed; however, in order to receive it, you need to ask for it, and, more important, believe you are worthy of its reception. How does Divine guidance appear in your life?

TRIAL

When Joan was asked during her trial if she had spoken with her Divine Guides while she was in captivity, she admitted that it took a while for her to hear her angelic messengers but that they did come to her. "Yes, both yesterday and today. There is no day when I do not hear them."

MESSAGE

I never admitted to anyone that when I was imprisoned, there were times when I was unable to hear my voices immediately every time I tried. This was very disturbing to me because I thought they had abandoned me. I was distraught and lonely, but the voices did return to offer support. Seek your personal Divine connections and ask your Divine Guides to make themselves known to you. Even if you don't feel that you are making connections with the invisible world, trust that your requests are heard and that you are not abandoned. These connections can be the source of your spiritual strength. Don't give up hope. You are worthy of Divine attention, and if you have faith that you will receive it, you will. This I can promise you.

MEDITATION

Close your eyes. Ask for a symbol of Divine guidance and let it enter your mind's eye and, more important, enter into your heart. Pay attention to the shape, color, or image that is being presented to you. When you have that image clearly fixed before you, ask your Divine Guides what you need to know right now, today. Don't be unnerved if you don't see or receive the message immediately; this meditation may take several tries and can be repeated as often as you like. Continue to send out the call to connect with the sacred realms and meet your Divine Guides, and believe in every fiber of your being that your request will be answered.

Flame of Courage 13

❖━━◦◉◦━━❖

VOICING THE EYES' WISDOM

The intuitive voices that Joan heard are available to you, and often these "voices" will speak to you through your own intuitive promptings. These promptings guide us, nudge us, advise us, and suggest solutions to our life's challenges if we take the time to listen for them. The fact that this wisdom does not stem from our rational mind does not diminish its value. The indigenous people of Malaysia believe that everyone has their own *med mesign*, or set of eyes, that allows us to see in various ways. Call upon your voices to help you connect with the wisdom that your internal eyes can see. Ask what your internal eyes can teach you about your illness.

TRIAL

Joan stated that she was not the only person who had the ability to receive wisdom from her voices and that other people chose not to see or hear them. When the court attempted to command her to renounce her claims that she heard voices (and saw visions), she announced fiercely: "If I were to be condemned and saw the fire lit and the wood prepared and the executioner who was to burn me ready to cast me into the fire, still in the fire would I not say anything other than what I have said. And I will maintain what I have said until death steadfast."

MESSAGE

My voices followed me; they guided me, no matter whether I was on the battlefield or at my parents' farm, in the king's mansion, or even imprisoned in a cell. These voices came to me often and told me not only what I needed to do, but how I could accomplish the seemingly impossible feats I was able to carry out. I believed in my voices above anything else, for they led me to and through my proper path. Your voices and inner prompting can do the same and lead you to comfort, peace, and healing. All you have to do is listen.

MEDITATION

Before you do this meditation, take out a recent photograph of yourself and study your eyes. I am sure you are familiar with the concept that the eyes are the "windows of the soul." During this meditation, you will be connecting with your soul source, which is your highest guidance. Once you can focus clearly on what your eyes look like, close your eyes and try to imagine your full face in front of you. Gradually, try to erase all of your features except your eyes looking back at you.

Once you see this image, imagine that you are looking past your own eyes and going deeper and deeper, to what is behind your eyes. Pay attention to witness and experience if you receive any insights, whether visual or intuitive. This is your soul source and above everyday experiences. You can think of this image as your soul self offering you the highest knowledge that can not only provide comfort and support, but also bless you with valuable insights about your healing path.

Flame of Courage 14

ETHICS

What is the ethical code you live by? When you are not in alignment with your personal ethical code, you may experience signals such as anxiety, agitation, or feelings that "this just doesn't feel right." How often do you ignore those signals? When you pay attention and listen to these prominent cues, you can easily access your inner knowing. When you have (and hold) faith in yourself and trust the message that something doesn't feel right, you are heeding the intuitive voice that is speaking to you. We all have the gift of this inner voice, and it is up to you to choose whether you want to respect it.

Make a list of the ethical qualities or values that you honor in your own life. This list is your ethical code. What qualities are most important to you? Kindness? Compassion? Truth? Are you kind, compassionate, and truthful with yourself? Are others? Insist that your healthcare practitioners reflect the attributes that are important to you and that appear on your list. If they (or others in your life) are unable or unwilling to do so, seek out physicians and specialists who share your philosophies and ethical code.

TRIAL

The men who interrogated Joan were purposely selected because they were all dedicated to her destruction. At that time, her popularity was legendary, and they knew that if they could convict her, then the legitimacy of King Charles VII would be called into question, which suited their political agenda. Out of seventy men who were chosen to be her judges, five refused to participate, on ethical grounds, because they knew that she was being used for political gain, and they bravely refused to have anything to do with her trial. One of these dissenters, Jean de la Fontaine, *"examinateur de la cause"* (examiner of the case), was so afraid of repercussions that he escaped to Rome. A man of integrity, he argued that the evidence in Joan's favor was suppressed (which it was), and he did not want his name associated with her conviction.

MESSAGE

I endured eight months of prison while chained to my bed. I was subjected to weeks of cross-examination and never knew what the inquisitors would do next. They tried to confuse me and make me admit I was lying, but I would not. I always believed in myself and my sacred mission to save France. Although few people publicly supported me, I relied on my resilience and integrity and my sacred path. You have a sacred path as well. Insist on having only ethical people on your life's journey because you have a choice. I did not.

MEDITATION

During this meditation, you will be creating a words-of-power statement that will reflect and have direct relevance to the ethical code that you choose to live by (see Flame of

Courage 3 on page 39 for an explanation of words-of-power statements). Take another look at the list you created for your ethical code and notice if any one word or sentence leaps off the page to meet you. Take your time. Using this word or sentence from your list, create a words-of-power statement that supports your commitment to honoring your ethical code and that feels right to you. The first thoughts that come to mind are the most authentic. You know you have the right words-of-power statement if, when you speak the words aloud or even think of the words, it reflects your truth. If you are unsure about what to say, you can borrow this statement until you are ready to fashion your own: "I will not abandon myself."

Flame of Courage 15

~◦━━◉━━◦~

FEAR

Fear is a valuable teacher. The belief that fear is always a negative state of mind and something to be shunned at all costs is a misunderstanding of the power of that emotion. Fear can make itself known consciously or appear unconsciously through the body's wisdom. It can manifest as a tangible feeling of dread, anxiety, or even panic attacks. The truth is that fear, though not a pleasant experience, is a valuable teacher. It tells us when we are out of sync. Fear can be a potent messenger and always has an important directive to impart. When you face your fears — when you name them, retrieve their wisdom, and transform them into knowledge — they won't hold power *over* you, but offer power *to* you.

Fear arises when we are feeling powerless and insecure. Those feelings can be greatly lessened when they are informed by wisdom. Fear at its core is often fear of the unknown, fear of what we have not experienced. If you can refocus your fear and use it positively, then it won't possess the same magnitude. Don't run away from these feelings and don't shut them down. Explore just where your fear is coming from. Find other people who have navigated their cancer journey to speak to about how they understand and work with their fears. Remember to only share your fears with those who truly know the energies of fear.

TRIAL

Because Joan feared that she would never be released from prison, she signed a "letter of abjuration." She was told that with her signature attesting to the letter's truth, she would be freed from prison. Unable to read, she didn't realize how damaging this letter was. The document stated: "I confess that I have grievously sinned in falsely pretending that I have had revelations from God and his angels." When she realized that she had signed away her integrity, she revoked her admission. Years later, at the request of her mother, the letter of abjuration was declared null and void by a papal court.

MESSAGE

I signed this document out of fear. I put my name on it because I was terribly afraid. I didn't know what to do, and I let others intimidate me. You do not have to let your fear rule you. You can examine your fears and give them the opportunity to speak with you. Once you understand your fears and their messages for you, which I did not, you will be able to proceed with full knowledge of both the dark and the light.

MEDITATION

Close your eyes. Try to locate where in your body the feeling of fear resides. Take all the time you need to focus on this fear with total acceptance. Don't attempt to push it out; just observe where it is. Once you have found its location, notice what color it is and what part of your body it chooses to hide in. Invite it to come to the surface, with full consciousness and acknowledgment. Once you have discovered your fear, speak with it and try to determine what wisdom it would like to share with you. By acknowledging your fear, and even welcoming it, you can allow the fear to be part of your healing journey. All emotions — even those that are not comfortable to experience — have a significant purpose. I assure you that fear can be a great teacher if you are brave enough to pause and pay attention to its message to understand and hear its teachings.

WILL

Your will is strong, like Joan of Arc's. A strong will can carry you through the most arduous of journeys even if it may not seem so at this moment. Imagine the gentle movements of a stream, which continues to flow regardless of the rocks in its way, because water has the intelligence to move around obstacles and take the path of least resistance. Your will can mirror the motion of the path of the stream when you recognize that all currents contain temporary blockages.

TRIAL

During Joan's trial, she was repeatedly asked about a "sign" she shared with King Charles to convince him that her message was indeed a direct message from God. Confiding in the king, she told him that she was the only person who could save France, and he believed her. The inquisitors attempted again and again to coerce her into revealing what sign she had shown the king to prove her Divine gifts. "I have always told you that you will not drag that out of me. Go and ask him [the king]. I will not tell you anything concerning the king: but that which concerns the trial…I will tell you. I will willingly tell you other matters, but the things I have promised to keep secret, I will not tell you."

MESSAGE

I refused to tell the court of matters that did not concern them. My Divine revelations were mine only and not to be shared. I respected my path and also recognize that my strong and unwavering will was the foundation for my strength and courage. Claim your unwavering will and belief in yourself because, I assure you, your journey is just as precious as mine was.

MEDITATION

Close your eyes. Try to imagine what your will looks like. Pay attention until one or more symbolic representations arrive. Then open your eyes and write down any words, or draw any images, that were received in your mind's eye. Imagine these symbols as your personal shield that you will carry with you during your quest for healing. When you are feeling overwhelmed and need help to navigate a challenging day, gaze at the words or images you have created — your personal symbols — to remind yourself that you have the necessary will and strength to persevere. Let these symbols become an integral part of you and know that you can retrieve them whenever you are in need. The message embodied in your symbols is private and personal, and you can be assured that it also holds great power; so keep it safe for yourself.

◆━━◉━━◆

CLARITY

Clarity is the key to balance — balance of your emotions and balance of the body. Clarity offers beautiful insights that are ever evolving because what your identified needs are at this moment will change in time. It is wise to recognize that your needs will be created and re-created during your journey. You have the ability to envision your path, understand it, and, most important, redirect it as your perceptions and intentions are altered. It is helpful, as a first step, to take inventory of all the elements of clarity, and lack of clarity, in your life. What are you absolutely clear about and would not change? Do you have sufficient understanding of your medical treatments? What would help you obtain clarity and direction? Don't be afraid to ask questions and to seek answers that will help you. Make a list of the areas that call out for greater clarity. Remember that not knowing does not indicate a flaw; it suggests that you are seeking a new direction and have not yet received the information necessary to move forward. Native American writer and artist Jamie Sams describes the voice of clarity as "the clear lake." Immerse yourself in this wonderful image as you create all the clarity you need at this time.

TRIAL

"And then she predicted to the King and others who were present four things that would happen. They did indeed happen thereafter. First, she said that the English would be driven away and thus the siege they had laid to the city of Orleans would be lifted and that the city of Orleans would be free of the English, but first she would send them an invitation to surrender. Next, she said that the King would be consecrated at Reims. Third, she said that the city of Paris would return to the King's obedience, and fourth, that the Duke of Orleans would return from the English stronghold. All of these things have come to pass."

MESSAGE

When I first set foot out of my childhood home to meet the king, I was confused. How could I possibly believe that I would have an audience with royalty? I knew I had to follow my destiny. When I first met with the king, I was a peasant girl; however, by the time I left him, I was commander in chief. I received clarity as I followed my path. Do not be disappointed if your clarity comes in small steps; it usually does. You do not have to know all the answers now — that in itself is clarity.

MEDITATION

Close your eyes. Focus on a particular situation that you would like to obtain absolute clarity about. Once you have that focus, let your mind clear completely and ask that the answers be given to you in a subsequent meditation, a dream, or a "knowing" that you will receive, accept, and can understand. Everyone is unique, and you may receive your information during your meditation today or during the days, or even weeks, that follow. All you need to do is trust that you will receive the information and keep an open mind and open heart. Just pay attention and allow yourself to be open to receiving answers.

Flame of Courage 18

PERSONAL POWER

True power has nothing to do with physical prowess. In reality, it derives from confidence and claiming your "right place" in the world. You may feel as if you have lost your power, but that is not true; try to reimagine instead that your power has been misplaced, because it is not possible for it to be removed. You can always retrieve it. When you are feeling unsure, unsteady, and hesitant, you have temporarily lost connection with your power. Personal power is both psychologically and spiritually based and is not power *over* someone else; it is a signature of self-mastery and of your ability to command your inner kingdom with grace and wisdom.

If you are feeling removed from your personal power, think about how often you give over your power to others. Do you give your power over to your healthcare providers without asking questions? Do you agree to a treatment, pill, or test that you know is not in your best interest? Are you willing to say no when something in your life or medical treatment does not feel appropriate? Do you agree to attend an event or be of service to another person when your energy is low or you would really like to say no?

When we betray our personal power, we *know* it, we *feel* it, and we *think* it. Reclaim your power by remembering when you gave it away and why. Who did you offer it to? Is this a familiar pattern in your life? Who told you that you were not entitled? Take your time to make this a conscious excavation.

TRIAL

"Whatever is going to happen to me, I will not say anything different than what I have already said to you. Truly, if you were to tear me limb from limb and make my soul leave my body, I would not say to you anything else."

MESSAGE

I followed the direction and guidance from my voices even though I was scared. I knew I had a mission in my life, and so do you. During the trial, I was bullied and confronted with every type of hostility, but I did the best that I could without giving over my power to those who attempted to control and humiliate me. Personal power is sacred and a gift that is held deeply within. Honor that gift and attend to your own internal calling. Personal power is not something that can ever be taken away without your authorization.

MEDITATION

We often give our power away to others — spouses, children, friends, colleagues, and healthcare providers — for many different reasons, especially to be "good" or to be loved. Women in particular, in an effort to please, often sacrifice their own beliefs and needs for the sake of keeping the peace. Close your eyes. Think about the last time you felt truly empowered and notice how you feel. After you have accurately recalled and relished every moment, shift your attention and remember the last time you gave your power away. Can you resurrect the way it feels when you give your power to someone else? Now ask yourself which is preferable. Repeat this exercise often to remind yourself that you are in control of your destiny and no one has the right, or your permission, to invade that personal territory.

◦━━◦━◦━◦

PRIORITIZE

Give yourself permission to put yourself first. Spend time doing the activities that have sacred value for you. Insist on arranging your life in a way that serves you. Prioritize by putting yourself on top. Choose healing words and actions, and encounters that bring you peace, and know — truly know from your core — that you can refuse to be drawn into chaos. You have a choice. Your journey into healing is dependent on your affirming that *you come first*. This affirmation of self is not selfish; it is necessary. Only you have the ability to change your life and re-create it in the way that supports you.

TRIAL

Prophecy predicted that a young girl, or "maid," would emerge victorious from the Burgundian and English battles, saving France and restoring its king to its rightful throne. History would have recorded a very different version of those battles without the unwavering passion and commitment of Joan of Arc. Jeanne la Pucelle (or, as her voices would later address her, daughter of God) was frequently challenged throughout her short life by those who thought her claims about rescuing France were ridiculous. She would repeat her favorite affirmation: "Have you not heard that it has been prophesied France would be restored by a virgin from the marches of Lorraine?" No doubt, when she repeated these words, it strengthened her resolve and was a strong reminder of her sacred quest. When she decided to devote herself to God, and trust her destiny and the direction of her voices, she did not relinquish her sense of self; she proclaimed her mission as liberator of France to reflect that sense of self. This was her priority.

MESSAGE

I believed in this prophecy with all my heart, and I knew that I had to surrender to the guidance I was given and that through this action of surrendering, I would achieve the goals that I was designed to accomplish. Once I truly understood that this was my fate and accepted it, I decided to make my mission, God's mission, the only priority in my life. I left my family and my former life behind. I did this because my will and God's will were the same. Put yourself first and decipher what your life's Divine mission is.

MEDITATION

Close your eyes. Imagine that your only priority right now is you and your quest for healing. Imagine feeling free, liberated and unencumbered by anything else. What would your life look like if you committed to yourself completely? What would that feel like? Allow the energies of devotion to self to inhabit your body. Pay attention to the feeling of surrendering to your needs. Try to memorize that sensation and experiment during the next week to see if you can bring the joy of release into your everyday life.

Flame of Courage 20

⊹⊱══◯══⊰⊹

VICTORY SPONSOR

Your victory sponsor is someone, or a group of people, that you have identified who can serve an important role in your healing and are willing to support, guide, and offer you solace when you are in need. Invite a victory sponsor(s) into your life to escort you through your sacred mission of healing. This person or group can include people you already know, people you wish to meet, or historical figures like Joan. No matter who you choose, your victory sponsor(s) should be people who truly embody the necessary triad of attributes for victory: courage, kindness, and compassion. Not only should your victory sponsor(s) be willing to commit to your healing process, but they also need to be willing to walk by your side, especially during the rough patches. Ask your physicians, your friends, or healers in your community to introduce you to people who can offer you guidance and serve as your sponsor. If you prefer to work alone with a historical figure who symbolizes victory, then visit bookstores or libraries and research the multitude of people throughout history who have been victorious in their lives. You can also discover your personal victory sponsor(s) through dream work, meditation, or visualization exercises.

TRIAL

Joan's voices were often accompanied by visions of Saint Michael, Saint Catherine, and Saint Margaret. "I saw them with my bodily eyes as well as I see you; and when they left me I wept, and I would have had them take me with them. Saint Margaret comforted me when I was wounded in the assault at the bridge fortress at Orleans." When she wanted advice on how to respond to the questioning during the court proceedings, they told her, "Answer fearlessly!"

MESSAGE

All of the saints who came to me offered me not only guidance, but also solace and companionship and support when I needed them, which was quite often. They were my victory sponsors and helped me travel through the difficult times in my life. Take advantage of the support you can receive from your victory sponsor. I can be yours.

MEDITATION

Close your eyes. Think about the importance of a victory sponsor(s) in your life and how that person or group of people could help you during your journey at this time. What could they do for you? Drive you to treatments? Take you out to dinner? Listen to your concerns and just be present for you? What would you like their role to be? Breathe and know that you can create the energy of support and compassion, and allow the image of a victory sponsor to come to you. Don't worry if you do not receive an image right away, but continue to ask that your victory sponsors step forward in your life. After you have identified the type of support you need, call upon your Divine guidance to assist you by creating opportunities for sponsors to cross your path. It may take a few active meditations to find them, but you can be assured that a victory sponsor will appear.

Flame of Courage 21

GIFT OF TEARS

Allow yourself to feel. Crying can be a soothing balm and a courageous act. It is a gift that you can offer yourself when you are feeling stuck, overwhelmed, or disheartened. Our culture often denigrates the act of crying. It is not usually welcomed and accepted; however, crying offers an opportunity for release that is a healthier expression of emotion than repressing what you truly feel. When you don't permit yourself to authentically feel, you may invite addictive behaviors — behaviors that often mask a deeper depression. Our bodies know the wisdom of tears and produce different chemical components for tears of joy and tears of sadness. In fact, our tears contain important immune enhancers. You are fully entitled to express your feelings, no matter how they appear to you or others. Remember that crying is not only therapeutic; it is also a strong and healthy response to stress. Always choose a safe place to cry and truly allow yourself to experience the healing that crying can offer you. You no longer have to carry around this burden on your psyche because you don't want anyone to think you are not strong. Crying reflects strength and courage. When you cry, you expand your capacity to reach deep into the painful places in your heart, and this, my friend, is a compassionate act. It is noble and not to be discounted. Will you allow your tears to reveal their healing properties?

TRIAL

The following is an excerpt from a report written by the Duke of Milan, who met Joan in Orléans: "Joan has great distinction.... She speaks little and shows great prudence in her choice of words. Her voice is soft. She has the gift of tears, and sometimes weeps abundantly, but as a rule she is smiling." The duke recognized the quiet nobility of Joan's tears, a recognition that might have been missed by many who believe the myth that crying is a weakness.

MESSAGE

I cried often and without worry that anyone would see me or judge me. I cried when I felt the need — before the king, in my jail cell, and in front of my men — without any shame. It gave me great comfort to cry. Don't be concerned with what you think others will say or think of you if you cry in front of them. My gift of tears was an integral part of my courage.

MEDITATION

Close your eyes. Imagine that you are surrounded by compassion and this compassion extends from the top of your head to the bottom of your feet. Compassion is available at all times and now envelops your being with a beautiful, luminous mantle of healing and protection, embracing your tears and sadness, and even your rage. You aren't alone. Invoke this veil of compassion even if you do not have support from the real world. Although you may not "see" the dimension of compassion, that does not mean it does not exist.

⤙═◉═⤚

INVITE THE LIGHT

When we are surrounded by light, we feel good, we feel energized, we feel healthier and at peace with our surroundings. Light has a long history of being used for its medicinal qualities. Historically, light therapy was practiced in healing sanctuaries physically designed to accommodate the sun's rays, in which patients rested in private rooms draped with cloths of various hues to promote healing. During the Renaissance, it was common practice for painters to depict saints and holy images with halos of radiant light, indicating enlightenment and connection to the higher realms. Light has always been a symbol of revelation and connection to the sacred. Creating the connection with your interior light requires being conscious of the spiritual domains, for light, by its very nature, is revealing and (literally or not) uncovers what is hidden from view. It is important to be willing to look at the dark places within to make room for the light to enter. Discovering your internal light, the light that provides connection to the spiritual domains, takes practice as well as commitment. It is courageous to create an internal space inside of yourself for illumination, even when your life seems covered with darkness.

Poet and singer Leonard Cohen beautifully wrote in his poem "Anthem": "Ring the bells that still can ring. / Forget your perfect offering. / There is a crack, a crack in everything. / That's how the light gets in."

You can invite the light into your life through active spiritual practices, ritual, and creating sacred space to allow the light to surround you. Clearing your home and mind of what is no longer needed is helpful for that illumination. You can choose to light candles that have scents you enjoy, arrange your bedroom as a sanctuary of peace and tranquility, or create a sacred ritual that will have particular meaning for you. There is no single prescription for direct access to the spiritual or Divine realms of light, so it is up to you to find the best way to enter.

The cycles of the moon are a wonderful visual analogy for the process of transformation. As the moon waxes and wanes, changing from full moon to new moon, it grows larger and more luminous, then recedes as it cycles through each passage. Note that during the waning cycle, as the moon becomes smaller, its glow can still be seen, before it returns to the beginning again. Allow the glow of light to create yourself anew, knowing that no matter how much light is visible today, it can — and will — change as you become able to bring more healing light into your life.

TRIAL

"The light comes before my voices. I am not going to tell you everything, for I have not permission, but I do say that it was a beautiful voice, righteous and worthy; otherwise I am not bound to answer you. There was a great deal of light [during the visions] on all sides, which was fitting. I rarely received revelations without there being the light."

MESSAGE

When I heard the voices, the light that enveloped me was from heaven. When I was inside of that light, I knew no greater peace and comfort. I bid you to invite that healing light into your own life to renew your spirit and nourish your body. Let Divine light lead you to peace and regeneration as it did for me — even in the most difficult of circumstances.

MEDITATION

Close your eyes. When you are ready, select a frequency of light that appeals to you — red, orange, yellow, green, purple, gold, blue, or pink. Imagine the color you have chosen entering your heart. Let the light sit in your heart and when you feel ready, watch as the light spirals up toward your eyes. Imagine the place between your eyebrows, often referred to as the "third eye," receiving the light and let it penetrate into your body, offering you healing. You will notice that the light slowly changes into a rainbow. Let its colors burn away all of your sadness, disillusionment, and confusion. Allow this process to continue as long as it needs to. When the process feels complete, imagine your healing taking place. See yourself feeling well, enjoying your family and friends, and participating in the activities of life that you love. Keep these images in your mind's eye, knowing that you can continue to work with these light images whenever you wish.

SECOND OPINIONS

Knowledge leads to wisdom, and the more knowledge you have, the better able you will be to make decisions that are important for your care and your healing. Although you may have a great deal of trust in your medical practitioners, it is wise to obtain a second opinion. Second opinions by experts in the fields of medicine (both traditional and integrative) can often provide you with new and unexpected directions for your cancer journey. Many women feel that if they seek a second opinion, somehow they are betraying their health-care providers; however, you need only be concerned with what is best for you. It is not offensive to seek other opinions; it is wise. Fundamentally, the best healthcare professionals are those who are confident in their abilities and have *your* best interests in mind — practitioners who are experts not only in clinical care, but in compassion.

Find out who the renowned specialists are in the field of medicine that pertains to your medical challenges. Don't feel shy about calling university research centers around the country to find out what types of research they are doing and see if any research studies are appropriate for you to take part in. Make sure you have all the facts about any research you might participate in, including side effects, length of commitment, fees, and, most important, the credentials of those who are leading the study. Find out how many people are enrolled in the study and who is funding it to make sure they have impeccable credentials and the study is in your best interests and not just the best interests of the researchers. Make sure you ask as many questions as possible before signing up for a research study that may or may not benefit you. Ask other people you know who have similar cancer challenges for referrals, read medical journals to help locate the professionals who may be conducting research that offers a different approach — perhaps an approach that can make all the difference in your treatment plans. You are not obligated to change your treatment plans; you are merely seeking information and education that can support your decisions, and those decisions are best informed by scrutinizing all options.

If you don't know who to choose for your medical care or are confused by the options, create a Comprehensive Treatment Plan. This plan can help you decide how to proceed. When choosing practitioners, it is always important to select experts who are knowledgeable about your type of cancer. It is also crucial to find healthcare providers whose clinical *and* interpersonal skills are excellent; one should not preclude the other. There are also people who specialize in guiding you through the maze of options ("hospital navigators" or "health advocates"), and you can take advantage of their advice.

Begin by writing down a list of all the practitioners who are part of your current treatment plan; next to each name, write down the advantages and disadvantages of working with them as well as their clinical experience. Do you have to wait in their office for hours? Do they look you in the eye when you ask questions? Do they return phone calls? Are they willing to explain terms or procedures you don't understand? Do you feel your opinions are respected and listened to? Select what is important to you when you are creating these lists. Create additional lists of experts you've identified who could provide second and even third opinions, and continue to add to these lists until you are satisfied. If you think about appointments with new practitioners as informational interviews, you can construct a framework in which you decide who is the very best for your healthcare needs. This is always appropriate.

TRIAL

Joan often consulted her voices to find out how to answer the coterie of inquisitors who daily interrogated and tried to confuse her. She was plucky, and although she was relentlessly challenged on all her beliefs, she consulted Divine guidance for revelations about how they wanted her to proceed. "What leads her to believe is the good counsel, comfort, and sound doctrine which she received from her voices."

MESSAGE

My voices were actually second and third opinions. When Saint Catherine, Saint Margaret, and Saint Michael came to me, I knew they could be trusted. Whatever I was going to do, I knew I could trust them because time proved their dedication and commitment to me. Ask for those second, third, and even fourth opinions — gather all the information you can so you can be empowered to make your decisions.

MEDITATION

I would like you to take out your Comprehensive Treatment Plan when you are ready. If you need more time to create it, that is fine; or if you would like to work with your partial list of current and possible future practitioners, that is also okay — whatever seems best for you right now. This meditation takes a little more time than many, so be sure to create uninterrupted sacred space. Center yourself and breathe gently in and out and try to release all worries from the day. After a few minutes, when you feel ready, look at your list of practitioners and say each name aloud, paying attention to your visceral response and the energy you are using or feeling when you say their name. Is your voice cautious? Loud? Comfortable? This will help you ascertain how you truly feel about your medical team. There is a message for you about each one.

If you feel that something is not quite right about a particular practitioner, then honor your internal feelings and keep searching for the right practitioner that feels right to you. Ask people you respect about who they work with and what their experiences are or were like. Decide what attributes are important for you: timely responses, compassionate care, attention and focus, innovative ideas for treatment, credentials, etc. You can change your list until you discover the right combination of healthcare professionals that you truly wish to have on your healing team, a team you are creating. Do not settle for including anyone on your list who doesn't feel right, and only choose people who you want to trust with your health. This is your right. Remember, it is permissible — actually quite advisable — to recombine your healing team until you feel safe and protected.

Flame of Courage 24

----※=◈=※----

INTEGRITY VOWS

Your integrity vows are sacred promises you make to yourself — *for yourself* — that can empower you when you are feeling alone and when everything is "too much." You are being reminded that you can build up your inner sustenance, a sustenance that you can easily reclaim by honoring your sacred vows to yourself. The courage to implement your vows is an art form and an honorable pursuit; however, before you can do so, you must uncover what may be holding you back from keeping your promises to yourself and following their wisdom. Can you write vows that are in accordance with the larger canvas of your life? Perhaps you have previously abandoned your promises to yourself because of a lack of hope or faith. You would be in good company — Saint Paul, Saint Francis, and even Mother Teresa experienced a lack of faith at some point in their lives.

When you think about your vows, pay attention to your first thoughts and allow them to surface, even if they contain a revelation about you that you don't want to look at. Refrain from judging yourself, because what you're receiving is just information — not right or wrong. Permit yourself to look at the barriers that keep you from honoring your promises to yourself so you can live in freedom from those restrictions. Your vows will reflect your highest ideals and possess dignity. Can you create vows that are in accordance with your highest good? In order to do this, you need to allow yourself to hold a greater vision for your life. It takes considerable courage to implement your vows and not just talk about them.

Have you ever abandoned yourself by not speaking up on your own behalf? When you remember that time, how did you feel about that experience afterward? What happened? Why did you choose that option? How could it have been different? Have you let other people take control of your decisions? Write down all of the instances you can recall when you have abandoned yourself. Once you have identified these times, take a moment and explore various alternative scenarios you could have chosen that would have supported you.

TRIAL

When Joan was asked at the beginning of her trial if she would tell the truth, she said: "You may ask me such things and to some I shall tell the truth, as to others, not....If you are well informed about me, you would wish that I were out of your hands. I have done nothing save by revelation....I don't know if you believe me but even if you do not believe me, I am sent from God."

MESSAGE

Faith and integrity were really the only things that I had to cling to. My integrity vows were dependent on adhering only to the guidance I received from the voices; these were the vows that I lived and died by. What vows will you commit to in your own life? What vows can you make today that mirror your integrity?

MEDITATION

Before you begin this meditation, take a moment and write a list of all the integrity vows you wish to keep in your life. When you are finished, look through your list and choose one of those vows to silently meditate on. Allow its message and its wisdom to be revealed to you. Do the same for each vow on your list, one vow at a time. This may take several meditation sessions over several days or weeks. As you go through this process, feel free to add new vows or delete any that don't serve you. You can return to your list of vows whenever you are feeling vulnerable and need support.

Flame of Courage 25

MAKE SWEEPING CHANGES

Making sweeping changes is not the easy route; however, it can be exciting. Some people thrive on change, and others find it quite difficult. If you find change very challenging, try altering your view of what change can be and you may be surprised. You are on a new and unfamiliar journey, and like all new journeys, change is at its core and is a requirement. As the explorer, you have the chance to step outside the boundaries of what you have known. It may be a daunting journey, but it can also be quite validating to seize control of more areas of your life. For example, if you have lost your hair, use this opportunity (yes, opportunity) to explore what it would be like to create a new image of yourself. If you always wore makeup, see how it would feel not to wear any makeup (but don't forget sunscreen). Experiment with your new image. Explore how you can use this new sense of self to your advantage rather than allowing the circumstances to use you. The magic does not dwell in the decision to wear or not wear a wig or makeup; the magic is in the acknowledgment that you are in charge of making the decisions.

When you have the time and the inclination, go through your closets and discard or donate anything you don't really like or feel good wearing. Get rid of all the clothes you have kept that are ill fitting or make you feel constricted. This is a chance to simplify your clothing collection and get organized. If you are in the mood to buy new clothes, then visit your favorite department store or a consignment shop that reflects your budget. Clothing choices you may not have considered before can allow you to reform your image — to paint a new picture that reflects who you are now. Bold colors, neutrals, or soft pastels can provide you with a new palette to stir a new life. Admittedly, change can be scary, but it can also be very liberating to create a fresh start.

TRIAL

Joan's choice to wear men's clothing was not only scandalous, but a primary reason for her undoing and at the core of much of the acrimony directed toward her. A woman who proudly dressed as a man, in full battle regalia, was unheard-of. Throughout her trial, her captors asked her again and again why she wore men's clothing. Her answers were both intelligent and brash. "The clothes are a small matter, the least of all things, and I did not take up men's clothes on the advice of this world. I neither put on these clothes nor did I do anything except by the commandment of God and his angels. It was absolutely essential for me to change my dress." She said that she "had done so because it seemed to her more suitable and convenient to wear men's dress being with men, than to wear a woman's dress." In fact, when she was asked about her "womanly duties," she told the court that there were enough other women to do them.

She acknowledged that she would be willing to "wear a long dress and a woman's hood" so that she could go to church during Easter, but she added the proviso that immediately after, she would remove the dress to put on male clothing. (Although she was told she would be given women's clothing to attend church, the clothing was never given to her.) She recognized that wearing male clothing offered her some protection from attempted sexual assaults by her captors. According to the principal notary of her trial, Guillaume Manchon, she complained that "one of the guards wished to violate her." Joan made her stance clear: "When I shall have done that for which I have been sent by God, I shall take a woman's dress."

MESSAGE

When I changed my dress from a woman's dress to a man's clothing, it not only changed the way I spoke, walked, and carried myself; it also changed something deep inside of me. I felt like a warrior — strong and confident. You can do the same.

MEDITATION

Close your eyes. Imagine yourself with a new image, perhaps an image you would never have previously chosen for yourself. Allow yourself to experience and visualize all the possibilities. Let these images appear without effort on your part. What do you look like? How does this image feel for you? If it doesn't feel right, say the word "delete" and move on. Once an image appears that excites you, think about how this representation can provide you with self-assurance and new insights. Remember you can alter this form whenever you wish. The physical appearance you create will often produce profound psychological changes, and those modifications can be beautiful. Take your time to explore how your new appearance can enhance your self-esteem.

Flame of Courage 26

NOURISH YOURSELF

Nourishment has many definitions; it can be in the form of physical nourishment, spiritual nourishment, or even emotional nourishment. What type of nourishment is missing from your life that you would welcome?

If it is physical nourishment that you have selected as your priority, investigate dietary changes that can enhance your healing. What types of food can offer you the nourishment you seek and also provide you with energy and vitality? Whole grains, fruits, and vegetables are always a healthy choice. Truly take the time to notice what foods attract you and can fulfill your body's needs right now. Visit farmers' markets in your community or ask a friend to bring you healthy foods that will not only nourish you, but nurture you. Ask friends or support group buddies to recommend a nutritionist who understands how to reinforce your healing and can help you create a health plan that is tailored for your individual needs. You may consider working with naturopathic doctors, homeopathic doctors, nutritionists, acupuncturists, or herbalists; however, make sure before you proceed that you have investigated their credentials, experience, and training. It is also worth your time speaking with others in your community who may offer you referrals to excellent practitioners in your area.

Read the medical literature so you are well informed. There is a great deal of research (called evidence-based research) on medical sites that can offer you additional information about integrative medicine protocols for people with cancer. PubMed (www.ncbi.nlm.nih.gov/pubmed), a respected website for research, is a rich source of information on the benefits and side effects of both mainstream and integrative medicine treatments in oncology care. There are many practitioners in integrative oncology care that are excellent, but I want to emphasize that it is important to research their credentials and training, because I want you to beware of working with someone who has limited knowledge or training. Always consult an expert and do not self-medicate. In addition, make sure you inform your physicians about any integrative medicine protocols you are using so they are aware of the impact these therapies might have on your treatment.

If it is spiritual nourishment that you need, imagine how you can bring spiritual sustenance into your life. Explore the possibilities — read spiritual books and biographies of people you admire, listen to inspiring audiobooks when you drive to work or run errands, and attend spiritual services you may not have considered before. Be open to the possibilities of nourishment that exist in your own backyard.

What type of emotional nourishment do you desire? Can you find that nourishment from family and friends? Visit support groups that may be held in your community, including Gilda's Club Worldwide or the Wellness Community. (Note that although Gilda's Club and the Wellness Community have joined forces to form a larger organization, the Cancer Support Community, some of the local chapters of these organizations have retained their original names.) Many spiritual organizations (such as synagogues and church groups) and yoga studios offer classes, lectures, and programs that may appeal to you. You might choose to work with a psychotherapist. If so, take the time to interview several to make sure the person you select to work with can offer wisdom from both head and heart. Don't be afraid to seek out the help you need. It is not a sign of weakness, but a sign of strength, to recognize that you need guidance. You may also consider speaking with spiritual directors, either those affiliated with your spiritual community or religious organization or those who work independently.

TRIAL

During the fifteenth century, it was customary for church bells to ring in the morning and at dusk, and Joan was a great fan of that tradition. As a child, she would often kneel in the fields near her home in prayer when she heard them ringing. She was so enamored with the tradition that, after a victory in battle, she ordered the local church bells to be rung while she prayed in the church. Perhaps her love of the bells stemmed from the fact that whenever she heard her voices, she also heard the sound of bells.

MESSAGE

I adored the sound of bells ringing, because I knew it would bring me solace and great comfort. Those sounds usually initiated contact with my beloved voices, the voices of nourishment for me. I urge you to find a sound you can use in your healing: Tibetan bells (tingsha), crystal bowls, drums. Reap the benefits of the healing power of sound.

MEDITATION

This meditation requires you to identify the particular type of nourishment you need in your life right now — physical, emotional, spiritual, or any combination of these. What areas have appeared in previous meditations? Make a list of resources in your life and community and identify what you are looking for — a nutritionist, masseuse, acupuncturist, spiritual study group, psychotherapist? Ask others to share their resources so you can add to your nourishment list. Share your list of resources so that others can benefit as well.

Close your eyes and in meditation, tell yourself that you will remember an important nurturing event from your life, from childhood or adulthood, that provided you nourishment. Don't try to force this; let it arrive of its own accord. Repeat this meditation for physical, spiritual, or emotional nourishment. A separate meditation for each category is essential so you can focus on each area individually. Once you have received knowledge about a particular type of nourishment you have experienced in the past, ask yourself how you can integrate that nourishment from your past into your present life.

—◦—

SECRETS

In all esoteric traditions, wisdom is respected, and secret doctrines are never revealed to the uninitiated. This is wise. If the seeker is not ready (either physically or psychically) for the revelations, secret knowledge can be misused or misunderstood, and even cause harm. Two of the necessary components for understanding yourself are truth and compassion. When you are reluctant to face painful truths, you deprive yourself of self-compassion — often because of judgment or blame. Are you completely truthful with yourself? Why or why not? How compassionate are you toward yourself? How can you bring more self-compassion into your life right now? What steps can you take?

TRIAL

"It seems to you, my lords and captains, that since I am a woman, I cannot know how to keep a secret. I tell you I am aware of all you have decided and assure you that I shall never tell what ought to be kept secret."

MESSAGE

I would like to tell you that the truth is contained in the secrets you keep close to you, and these secrets will also provide you great wisdom. What have you kept secret in your life, perhaps never even admitted to yourself, that is now ready to be revealed? Has your medical experience given you wisdom that you could not have received without going through this experience? Has it given you more compassion for yourself and others? Has it given you the ability to speak and recognize your truth, like me?

MEDITATION

Close your eyes. Ask yourself the following questions and through your meditation and stillness, uncover the truths by exposing your secrets to yourself.

> What secrets have you been hiding? Why?
>
> What would happen if you brought these secrets into your consciousness?
>
> Are you willing to explore your secrets without judgment or blame?
>
> What strength of character have you gained that you would not have had without your experiences with cancer?
>
> Can you take full credit for this strength of character?
>
> Would you be willing to think about how you could help others with your knowledge?

Flame of Courage 28

ARMY OF SUPPORT

Create an army of support for yourself and your healing. You are not expected to navigate your cancer journey alone. You are being reminded that you have an army of support behind you, although you may not be aware of it at this time. Make a commitment to build or acknowledge the army of support for your physical, emotional, and spiritual health. In addition to choosing the very best medical providers for your healthcare, make a list of people in your life who support you emotionally and spiritually — people you know you can truly count on.

If you do not have family and friends who are willing and able to rally around you when you need them, then create your personal reinforcements through your army of support. Don't be embarrassed that you need to do this; many people are not as fortunate as others who have the support they truly need and deserve. Call upon other people with cancer, join support groups, put yourself in an army of spiritually evolved people, and make choices about who you want in your army. Be discerning and make a list of people you *know* you can call upon when you need help.

TRIAL

"Although Joan was wounded in the shoulder from a cross-bow, she did not show herself to be wounded or leave the military action, but instilled such courage into her men that they leaped down after her in the moat, and using the ladders climbed up to the walls, forced an entry upon the English fort, and took the place by assault."

MESSAGE

I had men in my army who were willing to die for France and, if necessary, with me. They followed my lead and were available to support me at all costs. You are entitled to your army of support. Who will be in your army? Who do you choose to support you at all costs, knowing that they would be willing to catch you when you fall? Remember to choose wisely. Let me be the first person to join your army.

MEDITATION

Close your eyes. Imagine an army of support by your side and behind and in front of you. Envision a group of people, or perhaps a person, who really does "have your back," whether they are physically near you or not. Look deeper into the images of your army of support. The people who appear may surprise you. If someone appears in your meditation that you have not contacted, then this may be a signal to reach out to them and let them know you would welcome a connection with them. If you see images of those who are in the spirit world, then be sure to thank them for their help, knowing you can count on their assistance whenever you need it. You are being told that your army is just waiting for your signal to approach.

HEART REMEMBERING

The heart is a mysterious organ and has the extraordinary capacity to hold depths of love that often astound its owner. This muscle that keeps us alive also possesses exceptional recuperative powers, and because it is a muscle, it needs to be exercised on a regular basis. The acknowledgment of what love is and what it can be is integral to the heart's functioning, even when the heart breaks. There are gifts inside of the destruction. What does your heart remember? What and who have you embraced in your heart?

TRIAL

After Joan's death, her remains were thrown into the river Seine to prevent the crowd from stealing her body. Court documents reveal that her heart remained intact and was full of blood. It was believed that this was her final proof of the miraculous.

MESSAGE

Although my heart was frequently broken by the betrayals I experienced, I never gave up. I don't have regrets, for I believe I followed the path shown to me by my Divine messengers, although it was not an easy path to follow. I embraced my mission to save France with all of my heart, and I urge you to embrace your own healing mission with just as much surety as I did. My heart is a boundless vessel of love, and I am willing to share it with you whenever you wish. I remember you.

MEDITATION

Close your eyes. Think about someone in your life that you have not forgiven. Imagine their face in front of you. What do you wish to tell them? What can you do emotionally to release them? What would it take to grant yourself some peace?

When you feel able to do this (it may take several tries), tell them they are no longer needed in your life and do not have your permission to hurt you any longer. In your imagined conversation with them, tell them the truth of your experiences with them and that you have decided that their influence is not allowed in your heart or your body. Tell them you are now ready and *willing* to release all the painful associations you have carried, because you are on a healing mission. Be very clear that this is final. Remember, this exercise does not mean that you have forgotten what occurred, but rather that you have chosen not to be a prisoner to that pain. If, at a later time, you want to invite the person back into your life and heart because you believe they can enhance your journey, then you can always do so.

Take as much time as you need. When you are ready, try to locate the place in your body where their influence is, or has mostly affected you. Take a few minutes to scan your body. When you have located the area, imagine that you are holding a beautiful, glistening gold sword in your hands. Quickly bring your sword to the area where you've been connected to the person and cut the ties. In shamanic healing, this is called "cord cutting," and this sacred process allows the energies of someone who does not belong in your personal space (physical or emotional) to be removed. Holding the sword, bring your hands down in one swoop as quickly as possible and cut the cord.

Place your hands above the area where you cut the tie, and feel the energy of your body again. You should feel a change of energy, and you should also feel much lighter. You can repeat this process as many times as you like until you actually feel a difference. Then imagine a beam of white light in the area where you have severed your ties and fill that part of your body or mind with this light.

You may wish to document what occurred in this meditation. It is quite possible that your relationship to the person involved will be altered in the next few weeks, so don't be surprised if that happens. If you continue to feel that their unwelcome energies are near you, repeat this exercise.

-→≈◎≈←-

YOU ARE A HEROINE

You are the heroine or hero in your own journey. You are fearless, intrepid, brave, courageous, feisty, competent, kind, compassionate, and wise. You are the heroine that you seek. Remind yourself that you are the gatekeeper of these wonderful attributes and let them be of service to you. And remember that feelings of vulnerability and unsteadiness are an integral part of the journey of being a heroine; they are also beautiful, for they are part of what makes you human. All of your emotions will gain momentum, recede, gain momentum, and recede again — it is part of the path. You will move through all of it heroically.

TRIAL

Although Joan could not read or write, she frequently dictated letters to the English militia. Her command of language was quite advanced for a young girl who was illiterate.

She dictated this, addressing it to the king of England: "Surrender to the Maid, who is sent here from God, the keys to all of the good cities that you have taken and violated in France.... She is entirely ready to make peace, if you are willing to settle accounts with her, provided that you give up France and pay for having occupied her.... I am commander of the armies, and in whatever place I meet your French allies, I shall make them leave it....I am sent from God...to chase you out of all of France, body for body [every last one of you]....And if you do not wish to believe this message from God through the Maid, then wherever we find you we will strike you there, and make a great uproar, greater than any made in France for a thousand years."

MESSAGE

I could never have dictated such a letter if I didn't believe that I was the heroine of France, but I was on the heroine's journey. Don't doubt the capacities you have inside of you. I believe in you! I applaud your heroine's journey. Let me accompany you when you need me. I will walk beside you — heroine to heroine.

MEDITATION

Using the image of Joan of Arc for visual reinforcement before this meditation can be especially powerful.

Close your eyes. When you are ready, think about the concept of developing courage at this time in your life. In your mind's eye, place an image of Joan in front of you that reflects her courageous stance. Take time to study her demeanor, face, and body and try to imagine how the energies of her courage would feel in your own body. Let her interact with you. When you are ready, write down all that you have witnessed and experienced during this meditation.

CREATE YOUR OWN MANTRA

This Flame is without any prescribed text, waiting for you to identify the inspirational message that you need today. What words do you most wish to hear? The message can be on a theme you've been working with — such as peace, contentment, or wellness — or something different. You can create a words-of-power statement that has particular resonance for you (see Flame of Courage 3 on page 39 for an explanation of words-of-power statements) to use as the message or write messages to yourself that you wish others would say to you. Don't be shy: What do you really want to hear? Write out a few variations of the message or messages you've identified.

When you are finished writing out all the variations, choose one that you would like to work with in meditation. Write the message in your journal or on a card you can carry with you wherever you go — your car, your bed, your office, or even in your treatment room. Let this message be your personal mantra. Remember, the message is for you alone, so be truthful when you choose your words.

MEDITATION

This meditation is one that you design yourself. It may center on the mantra you have already created for yourself or another message of strength, or an image that appears as a symbol of courage for you. Allow yourself to meditate on this mantra, message, or image. Explore it deeply to obtain further wisdom.

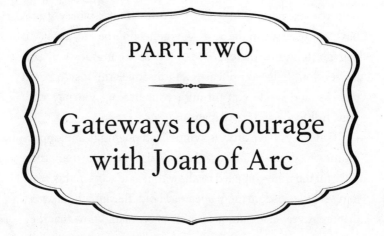

PART TWO

Gateways to Courage with Joan of Arc

This part of the book will provide you with tools to investigate, intuit, and access the strength, courage, and personal power you hold inside yourself. Remember that no matter what diagnosis you have received, *you are more than your illness*. I urge you to read this book for support during chemotherapy treatments, when waiting for a doctor's appointment, or when recovering from surgery or other procedures. You can use this book anytime you want to reconnect with Joan's courage. The guidance in the Gateways presented here will give you opportunities to discover how you can diminish your fears or feelings of helplessness. These Gateways will offer you a safe place to explore your journey.

The exercises you'll find in the Gateways were especially designed to reinforce and remind you of your own internal strength. These exercises include art assignments, guided visualizations, and writing exercises that work in tandem to help you excavate your internal world. (Don't worry if you have not used art in the past — you needn't be an "artist" to engage in any of the exercises.) These techniques will empower you, help you unearth and discover the insights you possess, and guide you through your healing journey with your full focus and participation.

Gateways have always symbolized openings and opportunities to cross from one place of significance to another. Take all the time you need to allow the Gateways in this book to reveal the wisdom these openings hold. Because the answers that are revealed are unique for every woman, know that they mirror your innate wisdom, a wisdom that has enormous therapeutic force. The cancer journey is challenging; however, inside those deep, dark moments of despair, strength and wisdom also reside.

The written word has always offered me solace and insight and clarity, and led me to my own internal wisdom, even when I didn't believe I possessed any such thing. But I have learned that when writing is derived from lived experience, it can always be trusted. The documentation of a woman's life, *your* life, is sacred. Everyone has their own story to tell, and that narrative changes daily. Allow yourself the time not only to document your unique narrative, but to help yourself discover your healing wisdom for the present and the future. In the Gateways, you will be encouraged to write down your thoughts and experiences, based on suggested meditations, writing exercises, or visualizations, without editing or having to write in a certain way. This type of "freewriting" allows you to circumvent your conscious mind in order to make connections with your intuitive mind. The intuitive mind has great intelligence; let your pen and paper lead you, and trust you will receive the information you need.

The sacred assignments in this part of the book will help you gain a deeper perspective into your own life and guide you to becoming the heroine of your own journey, with Joan of Arc's help.

How to Use the Gateways

There is no right or wrong way to respond to these Gateway exercises. Although each Gateway was written as a companion to the corresponding Flame of Courage in part 1, the Gateways needn't be used that way. Feel free to find your own way. Some days, you may find you have more energy and want to use a Gateway to delve more deeply into the theme you've explored in a particular Flame; other days, you may not be in the mood, and that is fine. Your sacred knowing will be waiting for your return.

You might choose to schedule a time during your day to work with the Gateways. If so, make sure you will be undisturbed during that time and if you need to, hang a Do Not Disturb sign on your door. This is *your* time, a time you can count on each day for an emotional, psychological, and spiritual retreat. One way to use this part of the book is to work with one Gateway each day for a month. If you opt for this approach, make sure you set aside sufficient quality time that will be considered your sacred space. If you prefer to work instinctively instead, you can employ the intuitive techniques explained in the introduction under "The Intuitive Process" and "Working with Intention" (pp. 23–26).

You may choose to work with other women or even begin your own healing group, using this book as your guide. I know from experience leading groups that the enormous power and velocity of energy generated by participants is very healing and can provide a safe sanctuary. I urge you to find others of like mind so all of the participants can share their accumulated wisdom.

Everyone has their own form, rhythm, gift of language, and artistic acumen. If you have an idea about how to work with an exercise in one of the Gateways, feel free to use your own idea and follow your intuition rather than the instructions provided for that exercise. If you find that you need more space than is available in your journal, you may want to purchase large art notebooks. These notebooks are especially helpful because they have plenty of blank space for writing and drawing. Don't worry about recording your responses neatly, and give yourself permission to make "mistakes." Also give yourself permission to "draw outside the lines" because it is usually when you venture outside the lines that creative wisdom appears.

Before working with any of the Gateways, take a few breaths. Shut off the phone and, if you wish, light a candle to sanctify the process. Rest assured that no matter what method you use, you can trust that you will receive the guidance you need at this time because *you* are making the choice with proper intention.

Gateway 1

～⚜～

VALOR

Take up your inner sword on your own behalf.

The following is a four-step exercise offering you the opportunity to discover your unique inner sword of valor. It is not necessary to complete the four steps in one sitting; if you prefer, you can go through each step on four separate occasions.

STEP 1: Write "VALOR = JOAN OF ARC" on a sheet of paper. Write it out as many times as you like. If you wish, experiment with different colors, using ballpoint or gel pens, Magic Markers, pencils, or calligraphy pens. For example, "VALOR" might be in red, and "= JOAN OF ARC" in other colors you select. If you are using different colors, notice which colors attract you. Feel free to create any type of designs around the words as well. Choose one of the designed equations that contains the colors you are most drawn to, and copy it at the top of a blank page.

STEP 2: Under the equation you wrote in step 1, write a list of times you recall when you felt full of valor. Once you have completed your list, choose one experience you listed that you would like to explore and put a circle around it. Write the following on a new page: "VALOR = JOAN OF ARC." Close your eyes and think about how you felt during the experience you circled. Did you feel strong? Proud? Brazen? Open your eyes and, on the page where you wrote "VALOR = JOAN OF ARC," write all the qualities that you remember you possessed.

STEP 3: Answer the following questions about the experience you explored in step 2 as authentically as you can. Write whatever comes to mind and don't edit yourself.

Who were the characters in your valor drama?

How long has it been since you felt the way you did during that experience?

What small steps can you take to honor, preserve, and revive that memory of valor in your life right now?

When you are finished, put down your pen and read aloud what you wrote.

STEP 4: On a separate sheet of paper, write "VALOR = JOAN OF ARC = [YOUR NAME]" until you actually believe it to be true. Write it as many times as you need to. Experiment with color and design if you wish. You may want to carry this sheet with you or place it where you can easily see and honor it each day.

Gateway 2

PATIENCE

It is not always a virtue.

Patience can also be viewed as calm endurance. Being patient, however, does not imply that you suffer needlessly. Imagine what it would be like to be released into a state of calm endurance no matter what you were experiencing. A state of calm is more than an emotion; it is an embodied state that you can feel inside your body and has weight and texture. Imagine a spiral. A spiral twists, curls, encircles — yet inside of its form is the circle, the center, or wholeness. You can create this sense of wholeness emotionally and physically. Trust the spiral of patience to lead you where it wishes to take you: up, down, sideways, yet always in motion. Your feelings of emotional equilibrium will be altered, and your sense of calm will change. The following exercise will help you gain personal insights into the feeling of calm endurance.

STEP 1: Write a description of what "calm endurance" means to you. Contemplate how calm endurance can speak to your life right now. When you are finished, review what you wrote and answer the following questions:

How can I discover this calm endurance?
What methods would I use? (Allow all possibilities
   to come forward.)

By activating the attributes of calm endurance that you have identified, you can begin to reclaim your emotional, physical, and spiritual stability.

STEP 2: Complete the following sentences:

I am calm when _____.
When I feel calm, I notice that my body is _____.
The last time I felt calm was _____.

STEP 3: The following visualization will direct your experience of calm endurance so that you can remember how it feels in your mind and heart.

Sit in a comfortable chair. Take a few moments and focus on the rhythm of your breath. Breathe in and out. Place your left hand on your chest and pay attention to the flow of breath in and out. Now imagine there is a movie screen in front of you at eye level. Visualize all the thoughts, words, and images from your day slowly appearing on this screen. Allow these things to appear on the screen as if you were watching a movie — your movie.

Notice how the screen gently dissolves into only white light. Enjoy this clear image of white light as long as you wish, and ask for a symbol reflecting calm endurance to arrive. Don't worry if you don't see anything right away; it may take a few tries, but you will receive this symbol, a symbol that is unique and especially for you. You may see an image, hear words, or see a color. Once you've received a symbol, open your eyes and write or draw it so you won't forget it. Be sure to document authentically whatever you experience.

STEP 4: Write the word "Patience" on a sheet of paper and place it in front of you. Respond to the following questions by immediately writing what comes to mind, without thinking about your answers:

What are my beliefs about the virtues of patience?

What are my beliefs about being *a* patient and about being patient?

What beliefs did I learn as a child about women who are impatient?

Are my beliefs about patience true?

What recent experience have I had that made me feel impatient?

In what ways was my impatience justified?

What happened as a result of my impatience? What am I willing to risk in order to speak up about my impatience? What issue concerns me at this time, and am I willing to be impatient or patient about it?

How can each choice serve me?

If I choose calm endurance, what can that teach me?

STEP 5: This step is especially helpful when you are making decisions about whether calm endurance is or is not in your best interest.

Think of a situation that requires you to choose between

calm endurance and speaking up. To help yourself choose, make a list of the advantages and disadvantages of each. This technique will help you understand and determine which choice can serve you. What can calm endurance teach you? Is this your best possible choice?

Use the symbol of calm endurance that you received in step 3 when you encounter situations that require patience. The more you examine the energies of calm endurance, the better able you will be to tell when it can serve you and when it cannot.

Gateway 3

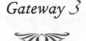

SURRENDER

Give yourself permission to surrender your self-doubts completely.

Although Joan of Arc is often depicted carrying her sword and shield into battle, it was her standard (that is, her flag) that carried the symbol of protection for her. Her standard reflected her commitment to the world of Spirit. Joan's standard was "sown with fleurs-de-lis, and showed a world with an angel on each side, white in color. The names Jesus Maria were written upon it and it had a silk fringe." During her trial, she said that she was "forty times fonder of her standard than her sword," and she carried the standard proudly as she led an army of twelve thousand men into battle. In this exercise, you will have the chance to create your own standard that you can use proudly as your healing symbol.

This exercise is a combination of writing and ceremony. Ceremony in Native American culture is a way to honor Spirit or the Creator. When circumstances in our lives are too overwhelming, chaotic, frightening, or out of our control, the best response, based on courageous wisdom, is to release the circumstances. This is not always easy, but it can be done. What I am suggesting is that although you cannot necessarily alter the problem, you can release the manner in which you respond to that experience. This exercise will help you give form to your feelings and provide you tools for surrender.

For this exercise, you will need one or more small (not full-size) flags in colors that appeal to you. You should be able to purchase them at a craft store. If you will be using multiple flags, choose different colors. For example, a white flag may indicate your connection with the Divine. A blue flag could symbolize your healing. A pink flag might help you work on issues of self-esteem and self-love. If you decide you would prefer to create your own flags, visit a fabric store and choose fabrics you can glue to a wooden rod to create your flags. You will also need colored pens that will write on the material your flags are made of, ribbon to tie around the flags, and any other item you would like to add to your flags.

STEP 1: Write down all the issues currently in your life that you need to surrender and that you are willing to surrender at this time. These might include such issues as pain, frustration, self-hate, anger, depression, and sadness. Make a complete and honest list. Don't include anything you think you should surrender but don't feel strongly about.

STEP 2: After you have identified all the issues you are willing to surrender, write them on one or more flags. It is your choice whether you want to layer all the issues on one flag or divide them among several. For each flag you are using, once you have written on it what you wish to surrender, wrap the flag tightly around its rod, bind it with ribbon, and set the flag aside.

STEP 3: Now you are ready to write a words-of-power statement that will help clarify your intention (see Flame of Courage 3 on page 39 for an explanation of words-of-power statements). Here are a few examples:

"I am willing to surrender my pain."

"I am willing to surrender my fear."

"I am willing to surrender my lack of faith in myself."

"It is released, and I surrender to the wisdom of God (or Spirit or the Creator) for the greater good."

These examples are only suggestions. Remember that your words-of-power statement should have a strong resonance with you and speak to your life's journey.

STEP 4: In this step, you will be offered ideas for creating a ceremony that speaks to your individual needs. Ceremony is an art form and includes the creation of sacred space through ritual and prayer. Ceremony is always holy and honorable.

When you have finished constructing your flags, you will need to decide where you want to place them. But first, imagine how you could use ceremony to call upon the sacred dimension. Your ceremony can include (or consist entirely of) lighting candles, saying your words-of-power statement aloud, using an altar you have created in your home, bathing, or simply washing your hands. Any of these can assist you in connecting with the peaceful energies of surrender.

Your ceremony can also include the process of burning sage, called "smudging." Smudging is a beautiful vehicle for creating sacred space, and Native Americans use sage not only to consecrate the space where a ceremony is taking place, but also to cleanse all of the participants entering that space. Sage holds great medicinal powers, and this pungent plant has been used for centuries as a healing agent. Its ability to remove any energies from our bodies or from the surroundings that do not belong to us is powerful and deserves respect. I agree with author Kenneth Cohen, who says that "sage is like a person whose presence is healing." When you use sage as a regular practice, you will notice subtle changes in energy — the energy of the room where you are smudging as well as your own energy. It is always a beautiful process. There are many good books on the art of smudging, and I suggest that you read about sage ceremonies before performing one if you are not familiar with the process. If you choose to burn sage, make sure you have air flow so you don't start a fire. You can also purchase a form of sage (an extract or liquid) that is prepared especially for ceremonial purposes if you don't want to burn sage.

If you will be smudging as part of your ceremony, light the sage and let it envelop you to cleanse your aura, the energy system that surrounds your body. Sage connects to the spiritual landscape, and in this case, you are the spiritual landscape. Allow the sage to surround your body — front and back, above and below. Don't forget to sage your feet. Healers use sage not only on themselves, but also to clear any unwanted energies from their medicine tools. After you have cleansed yourself with the sage, let its sacred power cleanse your flags.

When you have finished your ceremony, place your flags in a visible place in your home or sacred space. If you use smudging, you can always return to it whenever you feel that your energies are stuck.

Gateway 4

~⚜~

PRAYER

Choose a form of prayer for your healing.

There are many different types of prayer, and all are correct. Some people are more comfortable in traditional houses of worship, while others discover their source of inspiration in other activities and through creative acts, such as painting, writing, drawing, and dance, as forms of prayer. Whatever you deem sacred is your authentic form of prayer.

For example, one woman who was recently diagnosed with breast cancer told me she particularly liked using Saint Patrick's prayer, although she felt the need to change some of the wording:

Christ's light is with me.
Christ's light on my right hand.
Christ's light on my left hand.
Christ's light above me.
Christ's light beneath me.
Christ's light round about me.
Christ's light leads me toward my healing.

She said the prayer morning and night and told me she felt better equipped to face the challenges of her day when she incorporated this prayer into her daily sacred practice. Someone else might wish to adapt this prayer for their own use by substituting "Divine" for "Christ."

STEP 1: Light a candle in a sacred space in your home. Make a list of the important elements you would like to include in your prayer request — for example, elimination of pain, emotional and spiritual healing, or support from family and friends. Then write out your prayer. If you are comfortable with a prayer that you are familiar with and that provides you comfort, then use it. You have permission to change any of the wording so it reflects your personal needs at this time. If you prefer to compose your own prayer, make sure to weave your name and the important elements mentioned above into the prayer. Be as precise as possible. If you are not sure what you want to include, then you can borrow the following prayer, which other women have found helpful: "My prayer is that I will be in total harmony with all the healing energies that I need to bring me peace and freedom from pain."

STEP 2: Invite God, Spirit, or the Creator to accompany you in your prayers for healing. You may also wish to invoke Jesus Christ, Kwan Yin, Mother Mary, or Joan of Arc. I am particularly fond of Medicine Buddha and frequently invite his radiance into my prayer time. The spiritual power of prayer need not be confined to traditional religious figures, although you may address your prayers exclusively to one or more such figures if you wish. What is most important is that you choose a spiritual inspiration that is meaningful for you.

Gateway 5

~~~

QUIET YOUR MIND

Meditation offers you the opportunity to enter into the silence and an opportunity to make connection with your own internal wisdom.

Dedicate twenty minutes per day to an active meditation that you choose. You can begin by meditating for ten minutes a day, then gradually increase the length of time as you become more comfortable with meditation. I recommend that you use a meditation journal to keep track of how you feel before and after meditating. Each time you meditate, record the following in the journal: the date, how you feel before you start the meditation, and how you feel afterward. It is helpful to chronicle the differences you experience before and after meditation so you can document its efficacy over time. Using this type of meditation journal on a regular basis can also deliver unexpected insights.

The simple meditation exercise below can help you access healing energies for your body and soul, even if you are new to meditating. You can use this meditation whenever you feel anxious or out of sorts. It will help you quiet your mind and regenerate your body's chakra system. Your chakras are energy centers in your body that provide for a harmonious interchange between all the functions of the body. When your chakras need regeneration, you feel it, and the more sensitive you are to your body's messages, the more insight you will glean. If you are feeling unusually fatigued, irritated, out of sorts, or depressed, you can use meditation to offer vital healing energies directly to your body.

STEP 1: Sit in a comfortable position; if you're sitting in a chair, uncross your legs. Let your arms gently fall to your side or rest on your knees. Close your eyes and relax. Clear your mind of all distractions and simply breathe. Focus your attention equally on your breathing in and your breathing out. Continue to breathe. When you are ready, imagine a waterfall of shimmering white light above your crown chakra (see the diagram below). Once you can see the waterfall of light clearly, place yourself inside it. Let this shower of light flow from your crown chakra to the bottoms of your feet and permeate

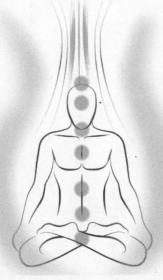

every part of your body. Allow the white light to gently probe any areas of your body that need healing. You may feel tingling sensations or a sense of peace. Stay with the white light as long as you need to.

STEP 2: When you are ready and have enjoyed the healing properties of the cascade of light, change the color of the light to green and visualize it flowing into your body. Imagine that each ray has direct access to every cell of your body. Allow the green light to penetrate deeply, offering extraordinary healing to and through you. Direct the green light to any areas of pain, knowing that the rays of light can offer relief. When you are finished, notice how you feel. Some women have told me that they felt warm and content, while others have experienced a much-needed boost of energy.

Gateway 6

TRUST

Trust your intuitive instincts.

Some women have the innate ability to trust their instincts, while others are not as comfortable doing so. However, trusting your instincts is a skill that can be developed. When you have an unwavering belief and confidence in your intuition, you possess a wisdom that can offer you extraordinary guidance. The more you trust your own visions and intuitive voices, like Joan did, the more solid and dependable your intuition will become.

STEP 1: Write your answers to the following questions, without thinking about what to write. Allow the answers to come forward without effort, in a stream-of-consciousness manner.

> What don't I trust about myself?
>
> Who told me that I couldn't trust myself? Is this true?
>
> What could happen in my life if I learned to trust myself and my intuitive voice?

STEP 2: When you are ready, read what you wrote. If you find that you have documented issues from your past (or present) involving someone who told you that you couldn't be trusted, write a letter to that person. (This letter is for you alone and is not meant to be mailed. However, some women have actually mailed a letter to the person they were addressing and have found it quite therapeutic, though obviously you would not mail a letter to someone who you think might be a danger to you or your family.) In the letter, explain that what they said is not true and that you will not allow their opinion to influence your life any longer. If you discover that *you* do not trust yourself, write a letter to yourself once you feel *certain* that you can trust yourself. You may find through the process of writing this letter that you gain extraordinary insights. Whoever the appropriate recipient of the letter is, if you are unable to write it at this moment, that is fine; just put your notes aside and return to the exercise in a few days. Record in your journal any names that came up so you won't forget your insights.

Gateway 7

━━◦❦◦━━

STRENGTH

**Your internal strength is just as valuable
as your physical strength.**

Physical strength is important when you are facing a cancer diagnosis or any serious illness. During the course of your treatment, you may not be able to participate in the same activities that you previously engaged in, but that does not mean you cannot find pursuits that will help you regain your strength. You can rebuild your strength and slowly add increasingly challenging activities as your stamina returns. This exercise will also help you take inventory of your beliefs about emotional strength and identify any blocks that may be holding you back from gaining full possession of your internal strength.

STEP 1: Write down all the activities that come to mind when you think about restoring your strength. For example: walking, yoga, stretching, swimming, tai chi, bike riding, or lying on the floor inviting the energies of your breath to guide you to internal balance. Among the activities you've listed, identify those that you genuinely enjoy and that you can do right now. Then choose one activity that you are willing and able to commit to do on a regular basis. Schedule this activity as you would any important meeting with your healthcare team, because physical exercise (even gentle exercise) is an important component of your healing.

STEP 2: When you are ready, write the answers to the following questions:

> What words describe emotional strength for you?
> What are your beliefs about your emotional strengths?
> What does "too emotional" mean to you?
> Can you find the wisdom in being "too emotional"?

Take time to write down a list of everything that comes to mind when you think of your emotional strengths. When you are finished, look at your list and write everything you can think of that supports the points made in your list. Include actual experiences in your life when you felt emotionally strong. For example: "I believe that emotional strength means the ability to go on, to tackle each day of my recovery as best I can. When I came home from the hospital after surgery, I realized just how strong I was."

Now take a moment and think about how you feel internally, inside of your body, when you are emotionally strong. Describe in writing what it feels like. For example: "My body feels centered and focused when I am emotionally strong. I am able to function each day, to take good care of myself. I sleep better, my body feels more at peace, and I am without internal emotional chaos."

Complete the following sentences to probe deeper:

Emotional strength means _____.

I felt (or feel) emotionally strong when _____.
When I am emotionally strong, my body feels
_____.

Retrieve this exercise whenever you feel that your internal or external strength is unavailable. Use this writing exercise again and again to remind yourself that *you do* possess emotional strength — you only need to reclaim it.

Gateway 8

~~~~~~

HUMOR

Humor is a deflector of negativity.

In the corresponding Flame of Courage, I suggested many ways to integrate humor as a shield against negativity, and provide opportunities for protection from negative beliefs or worries you may be experiencing. In this Gateway, you will learn techniques for creating a visual shield that can provide you with protection from those negative beliefs. These beliefs can manifest as self-doubt or you may be surrounded by people who are not in true support of your healing journey. Warriors throughout the centuries have used shields both for protection and to display their wartime affiliation. The symbols that the shield portrayed were often designed to reflect personal emblems. It was not unusual for the warrior to perform ceremonial actions before battle to invoke the invisible properties of security that their shields contained and were awaiting release. The symbol depicted on their shields had purpose and sacred power.

During this exercise, you will be creating your own shield of protection, both for a personal display of courage and as a deflector of negativity. It doesn't matter if you have had artistic experience or not; what matters is that you choose symbols, words, and colors that have meaning to you.

STEP 1: Think about the word *shield*. Write down any words, and draw (or cut out of magazines) any images, that come to mind. Write the words in your journal in a favorite color. Put the images aside. Close your eyes and concentrate to see what images or words appear to you. Write down or draw any words or images that you have seen or heard. Pay attention to any colors that may have appeared in your image. Although colors can signify many different things, some of the possibilities include the following: pink can represent protection; gold can represent armor; red can represent fierceness; white can represent clarity; purple can represent Divine assistance.

STEP 2: You will now create your shield. You can choose to draw your shield on paper, a piece of cardboard, or a paper plate, or even create a sculpture out of clay if you wish. The size of your shield does not matter, and you can choose what you like. As you create your shield, you can draw or design it based on the images you have received in meditation or choose images that are absolutely authentic to your own spirit. You can also include words that have a strong force and speak to you. If you wish, you can continue to collect any images that you connect with from magazines to create a collage on your shield. You may wish to draw the outline of a shield and glue the images inside of that outline. Please note that the shield you create does not have to be in any traditional form. One woman imagined her shield in the form of sparkling pink light that she "wears" through visualizations each night.

If you've created a physical shield, place it near your

bed, in your office, or inside your date book, to remind you that you are "shielded" from any less-than-positive encounters. Joan of Arc's shield was white light, a healing light from her voices that she "wore" all the time. This was her Divine armor.

Gateway 9

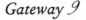

COURAGE

***Let your courage lead you to
solid and secure ground.***

This visualization exercise will teach you how to identify
your Courage Guides. Joan relied on her voices and spiritual
encounters. You too can discover your own Courage Guide
to assist during your healing journey.

STEP 1: In this step, you will have the opportunity to connect with your Courage Guide, and this Guide can offer you
healing and connection whenever you wish. This meditation
is also quite relaxing and an opportunity to blanket yourself
with the healing energies that your Guide can offer you, especially when you are having a difficult time. It is helpful to
make an audio recording of the meditation so you can listen
to it while meditating or to have someone read the meditation to you.

> **MEDITATION.** Close your eyes. Release all thoughts
> of your day. Relax. Breathe in and out, and when you
> exhale, release any thoughts that may be troubling
> to you at this time. Put those worries and concerns
> into an imaginary bubble and send it off into the sky

like a balloon. Watch it rise up, up, up until you can't see it any longer. Listen to the steady rhythm of your breath...in and out...in and out. Imagine you are in a beautiful setting — a mountaintop, a grassy meadow filled with lavender flowers all around you, or perhaps by the ocean. Enjoy where you are.

You are going to meet your Courage Guide — someone who has a message for you. Look up, and you will see them approach you. It may be someone you know or have known in your life, or it may be someone or something totally unexpected — an animal, a color, or a whispering of communication. If you don't recognize who or what you are seeing or hearing, then ask them to introduce themselves to you.

Your Courage Guide has something to give you. Hold out our hands to receive their gift. It may be an object or a message that will have meaning just for you. Just pay attention. After you have received this gift, thank them. If the gift is an object, take a few minutes and when you are ready, look at it; if it is enclosed in something, open it up. The gift may also be Divine words whispered only to you. Ask your Courage Guide if they have any other information to offer to you. You can ask them how to connect again in the future.

Open up your eyes and return from this meditation.

Once you have completed the meditation, write down everything you saw, experienced, and received from your Courage Guide.

STEP 2: Take out a blank piece of paper and draw the image of your Courage Guide as clearly as you remember it. You can also add your Courage Guide's name, any messages you received, and a verbal description or simple drawing of the gift you were given.

When you are feeling less than courageous, review your notes from this exercise for support.

Gateway 10

꠸글

COMMEMORATION

Take stock of who you are.

Taking stock of who you are is not an easy process and may be time consuming, but it is important to do. All too often, we forget who we are and minimize what we have accomplished, which in turn negates our successes and damages our self-image. When you believe that your accomplishments happened by chance, or through others, you are not entirely correct — without you, the constant in all the situations, your achievements could not have occurred.

STEP 1: Write down all of the accomplishments you have achieved in your life, no matter how large or small they appear to you. Resist the impulse to judge these accomplishments in terms of merit; just write what comes to mind. It is helpful to list these achievements by age, as follows:

Age 1–10: List of your accomplishments
Age 11–20: List of your accomplishments
Age 21–30: List of your accomplishments
Age 31–40: List of your accomplishments
Age 41–50: List of your accomplishments
Age 51–60: List of your accomplishments
Age 61–70: List of your accomplishments

Age 71–80: List of your accomplishments

Age 80-plus: List of your accomplishments

When you are finished, read your list aloud and keep this list with you so you can remind yourself of your life's accomplishments.

STEP 2: Write down all the activities you have always wanted to do but never took the time to pursue. Only list activities that you are energetically, physically, and emotionally capable of doing. Here are some suggestions:

- Visiting an orchid garden
- Going to lunch with a favorite family member or friend in a beautiful café
- Going to a movie by myself
- Taking a quiet walk in the early morning hours
- Buying a paint-by-number set
- Knitting something for a special friend
- Writing in my diary or reading my old diaries
- Coloring
- Buying flowers every week at my favorite flower shop
- Sitting by the sea and simply inhaling the air
- Visiting museums
- Taking photographs of inspiring images

Look through your list and remove anything that doesn't truly call to you or that would be difficult to accomplish at this time. Choose *one* activity and put it on your calendar so it becomes a part of your schedule, as further commemoration and celebration of you.

Gateway 11

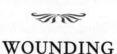

WOUNDING

Seek the wisdom contained in the wound.

When we think of the word *wound*, we usually do not associate it with sources of wisdom or personal power, but your wounds can reveal great knowledge and self-understanding. You may know people who have shown you their scars from war, battles with cancer, or life's circumstances. When someone offers this visual illustration to you, it is an honor to be part of this connection with them. Revealing one's wounds shows courage, and wounds survived are a badge of honor. Your wounds are sacred, and I urge you to acknowledge the power — yes, power — inherent in your wounds, for in my experience, that acknowledgment is formidable and never leaves you. The following exercise is not an easy one but has its rewards.

STEP 1: Write the following headings in your journal (leave some space for writing under each one): "Mind," "Body," "Spirit." Underneath each of these headings, list all of the woundings that you feel in that area of your life. Be honest with yourself. If you find that you can only write one or two woundings, that is fine; just return to this exercise as many times as you need to, until you have completed your list. If you wish, you can go to the next step even before you finish the list.

STEP 2: Now you will use writing exercises to work with each wounding you listed. For each wounding, ask yourself whether it is really true for you and what messages it might hold. For instance, if under "Mind," you wrote, "Lack of emotional security," take some time to think about whether this perceived lack of emotional security is true for you. Then ask yourself this question: If I allowed the lack of emotional security to speak with me, what would its message be? The following is an example:

> **WOUNDING:** I feel emotionally unstable.
>
> This feels true for me now, but I don't remember feeling this way my whole life. I began feeling unstable after my diagnosis.
>
> My emotional instability is telling me that I need to be taken care of, that I need to share my feelings of vulnerability and ask for emotional support from my family and friends right now.

Take as much time as you need to engage with this dialogue for each of the woundings you have listed. The key to this exercise is to listen to the message contained in the wounding. This exercise may bring up emotions and memories of the past, and that is okay; take your time to examine your woundings with respect, for they are an integral part of you. And if you find that you need additional support from a professional, then do not hesitate to reach out.

Gateway 12

DIVINE GUIDES

Seek out guidance from a Divine source.

Everyone has Divine Guides, or a Divine Guide, although you may not be familiar with the concept. Think about a time during your life when you knew you were somehow divinely guided — perhaps it was when a magical door opened and you received your perfect job, met your husband or wife or partner, or discovered the perfect solution to a serious problem. Usually, when these synchronicities happen, there is no effort on our part. We often use the word *coincidence*, or even *miracle*, to describe these occurrences. The answers seem to appear as if out of nowhere, but I believe that these moments are indeed divinely guided.

This exercise includes dream work to help you get in touch with your Divine Guide. Dreams can be a powerful source of insight. I have received profound messages through my dreams. When I was in the midst of writing the book *The Way of the Woman Writer*, I was given a beautiful quote during a dream, but I was so caught up in my sleep reverie that I almost missed it. However, the message grew louder and demanded that I write it down, so I followed its directions. The words I was given were so lovely that I used them as the dedication in that book.

STEP 1: Document in your journal everything you can think of in your life that you could not explain and that seemed divinely guided. Explore your memories of childhood, young adulthood, and adulthood. I assure you that everyone has had these gifts during their lives.

STEP 2: This step will help you make contact with your Divine Guide through dreaming. Put a notebook by your bed so that, on awakening, you can write down any information you've received during the night. Before you fall asleep, while you are still in the "twilight zone" between sleep and aware consciousness, tell yourself that you will meet your Divine Guide in tonight's dream. Ask your Divine Guide to come forward. You may have to repeat this request nightly until you receive a response. Please don't give up — you can and will meet your Divine Guide through your dream work, but it is not unusual for it to take many weeks, or even months. I assure you that even if you don't usually recall your dreams, you can learn this skill. This remembering of your dreamscape not only requires practice; it also requires trust. Trust that your connection to your Divine Guide will indeed take place. Your Divine Guide may appear in a multitude of ways: as a person, color, message, or even an animal. It is important not to discount "how" your Divine Guide may appear but allow your Guide to make connection as they choose to arrive. In addition, it takes commitment because it is an active, cocreative process: you will be working intently with the images, dialogue, textures, and feelings of your dreams just as you would engage with the "real" images and characters of your daily life.

Dreams have a unique language that is symbolic, and it may take some time to decipher their codes. Pay attention to all of the wisdom you obtain, including all the details. Inside those very details and within the fragments that you remember, you can uncover valuable clues to assist you in meeting your Divine Guide.

If you decide to delve deeper into your dream world, then you need to cultivate an atmosphere of receptivity. You can set the stage for dreaming by taking time to unwind before you go to sleep, taking a bath, reading, or conducting a ritual that signals to you that it is time for sleep. When you wake up, before you even get out of bed, pull out your notebook and write down or draw any images, words, or narrative you remember. Through practice, you can retrieve the memory of your dreams by reminding yourself, before you fall asleep, that you will write down everything you recall on awakening. You may also be awakened during the night with images or messages; and even though it is hard to maintain enough discipline to do so, it is important to document these images or messages so you won't forget them.

You might also wish to keep a dream diary that you write in while fully awake and where you document in greater detail the insights you receive. A dream diary will allow you to make an even more significant connection with your Divine Guide. You can also use a tape recorder left by your bed to record your dreams, but it can be difficult to use when you are dusted with sleep. The recording of dream narratives, whether in audio or written form, is sacred and can become a thoughtful practice. Regardless of how you document your dreams, you can record how your dreams feel somatically, by taking an inventory of how your body responds during or after your dreams. You may have dreams that depict what is happening inside your body, for the body holds wisdom long before it reaches consciousness. This information can often suggest therapeutic possibilities, for both your physical and emotional well-being, that you may not be aware of or provide you messages about how you can heal.

When you have met your Divine Guide, don't hesitate to ask for assistance, for dream healing is a spiritual process. Joan knew that her voices would provide her with the guidance that she needed, and so can your Guides.

～⟫⟫⟫⟫～

VOICING THE EYES' WISDOM

Clarity from different perspectives.

According to the indigenous people of Malaysia, the *med mesign* is the conduit for allowing us to "see" from a different perspective. This Gateway will help you access the inner meaning of your internal eyes, or *med mesign*, described in Flame of Courage 13. This ability is not usually explored unless you have studied metaphysics or have an ongoing spiritual practice. My interpretation of this concept is that through connection with our heart self, or soul self, we can obtain the clarity to "see" inside of ourselves, and this ability offers greater self-reflection. Although I am not referring to the ability to literally look into your body as medical intuitives can, I am suggesting that you can "see" inside of yourself by using art and meditation. The steps below can guide you toward looking deeply within to explore and to access your individual intuitive voice. You will not only design a new set of eyes, but you will also receive the wisdom those eyes contain.

For this exercise, you will need a set of Magic Markers, colored pens, or colored pencils and a recent photograph of yourself. Pick a photograph where you can see your eyes clearly and distinctly.

STEP 1: Place the photograph in front of you and draw the eyes that you see in it.

STEP 2: Next, look at your photograph and your drawing, and write all of the words that come to mind to complete the following sentence: "My eyes are in direct communication with me, and they are revealing _____." When you are finished, put your drawing and your notes aside.

STEP 3: Repeat steps 1 and 2, but this time, change your drawing to reflect how you would like your eyes to look. For instance, you may wish your eyes to show a person who is at peace, has more vitality, or is happier. Ask yourself what inward state you wish your eyes would reflect.

STEP 4: Close your eyes and clear your mind. Envision a screen in front of your eyes that can remove all troubling or random thoughts. Keep your eyes closed and pay attention to any images you see. Ask to see your personal set of "internal eyes." These internal eyes have a message for you and can reflect your soul. Wait to receive the message, which may be verbal or a visual symbol.

STEP 5: When you are finished, draw or write down any images or messages you received. Don't be surprised if the eyes you saw in your meditation are not familiar. Just honor whatever images appeared to you.

STEP 6: Complete the following sentences in your journal:

My internal eyes have the following qualities: _____.

My internal eyes are a guide bringing me information for my healing. The message I received from them was _____.

When you are finished, take some time to look at the designs you have drawn, as well as the text you have written, for each step of this exercise. Now put each of the images you have drawn in front of you. Compare the texts for each step with the images for that step. Listen to the narrative you have created for any insights. You may choose to repeat this exercise periodically, for it is a potent one.

Gateway 14

~~~~~~

ETHICS

What is the ethical code you live by?

Think about the word *ethics*. It is often defined as a "system of conduct or behavior." In this exercise, you will have the opportunity to invent your own system that you can live by each day.

STEP 1: Complete the following sentence in writing: "My ethical code contains the words _____."

STEP 2: When you have finished your list, create your ethical code by using the words you selected. This will make that code more authentic and one that speaks to you so that you can live your life in alignment with the qualities you value.

STEP 3: This step will enable you to design an ethical code that you wish to experience with the members of your healthcare team, your healing team. You may want to give it a name that has meaning for you. Make a list of all the attributes that make up the ethical code that you require your healthcare team to abide by. This list may be similar to your own ethical code, or it may differ. Of course, you cannot change other people's behavior, but you can insist that *your* healthcare practitioners possess qualities similar to those that you have identified as important in your healthcare ethics code. For example, your code may emphasize compassion, kindness, knowledge, and expertise. If you would like to borrow the following code until you are able to create your own — feel free to do so: "I expect to join forces with my healthcare team who embody excellence in mind, body, and heart."

STEP 4: Review your healthcare ethics code. It is helpful to consult this code when you are having second thoughts about working with a particular healthcare professional. Remember that the people you select for protecting you during your cancer journey are joining forces *with* you to create the optimal treatment plan for your healing. Intrinsic to the delivery of this plan is the expectation that it will be communicated with kindness.

Gateway 15

~~~

FEAR

Fear is a valuable teacher.

The word *fear* has been given a bad reputation although it is a valuable teacher. Feeling fear is uncomfortable and sometimes quite terrifying, but it does serve a purpose. That purpose is to make sure you are paying attention to its wisdom. Fear protects you and tells you that you are in danger, and anxiety is often the cloak of fear. One of the best ways to access your fears is to invite them into your consciousness, bringing them out of the hidden realms so their ability to overpower and frighten you lessens. Once you do so, you are on equal footing with your fears. In this exercise, you will be invited to write them down, no matter how difficult this may be. By naming your fears, you acquire perspective and have the chance to educate yourself about how fear can be a welcome messenger.

STEP 1: Write the heading "My Fears" at the top of a page in your journal. Under that heading, make a list of all of the things you are fearful of. Be honest and don't hold back. List even the deepest fears — those that you perhaps have never given voice to or have never given yourself permission to voice.

STEP 2: Look at your list and see which fears are reality based and which ones were instilled in you by someone else and do not belong to you. Next to each fear in your list, make a note indicating whether the fear is your own or someone else's fear that you are carrying. For each fear, ask yourself, "Who owns this fear? Does it belong to me?" List the name of the person who owns the fear.

STEP 3: When you are ready, write a letter to each and every person who appears on your list whose fear you have chosen to carry inside yourself. Yes, you have chosen to carry their fear, and you can easily discard that choice. Don't worry — you will not be mailing this letter, and you will not be asked to confront anyone with the contents. This exercise is for you alone. The more honest you can be, the better, because this inner work can promote your healing.

In your letter, include how the other person's fears have manifested in your physical, spiritual, or emotional life, and what price you have paid for these fears. At the end of the letter, include a statement that you are now ready to release these fears and won't carry them any longer. When you are done, I suggest that you don't read the letter, but crumple it up and toss it in the wastebasket; or you can burn it and toss the remnants into the ocean or a nearby lake if you have access to one.

STEP 4: The last letter you will write is a letter that helps you address your own fears. You will name and chronicle how your fears may manifest inside your body or how they are affecting you emotionally and spiritually. In your letter, also cite examples from your past that exhibit your success and fearlessness. By virtue of your experience with cancer, your courage is commanding. Here is an example of one woman's writings about her own fear.

> [*Description of fear*] I am fearful of the unknown, and whenever I don't know what is going to happen next, I feel immobilized and can't get out of bed.
>
> [*Response to the fear*] Although I don't know what is going to happen next, I know that I can ask other people who I trust and who have been through cancer treatments. I can ask them to tell me what they experienced so that I am not afraid. I can use this information to empower myself. I have been frightened of the unknown before, when I went away to college, when I began my new job, when I went through my divorce and resurrected my life. And I was just fine.

When you actively dialogue with your fears, then their ability to continue to cause harm is destroyed. Engaging in a conversation with this emotion (or any emotion), and naming and identifying those fears, can be quite illuminating.

Gateway 16

❧❧❧

WILL

Your will is strong.

A strong will is required when you are facing any type of challenge in your life and is particularly important to possess during your journey with cancer. I find it interesting that often the idea of a "strong will" or being "willful" not only challenges our self-perceptions but often is seen by others as problematic. Others are not always supportive of this personality trait, especially in females. Women are often discouraged from being "willful," and it is viewed as a negative trait; yet for men, this trait is celebrated and curries respect. I want to remind you that your will is not only strong; it is beautiful and welcomed. Joan of Arc supports your "will."

STEP 1: Write the words that come to mind when you think of what you wish to achieve using your will.

STEP 2: Write what enters your mind when you remember what you have willed in the past.

STEP 3: Make a list of all the challenges you can remember facing when you've tried to assert your will.

STEP 4: Select one word or phrase from each of the three categories created in the previous steps. When you have completed that process, write one or more sentences of support to empower you to assert your own will now. Be sure to create one or more sentences that combine your experiences, both positive and challenging, so you can see how you were able to work with your will successfully. For example, one woman wrote the following:

> What I wish to achieve using my will: Self-reliance. Healing. Ability to think positively.
>
> Things I have willed in the past: Going to college on scholarship. Meeting my partner. Moving to a beautiful home.
>
> Challenges to my will in the past: Lack of family support. Losing my job. Illness.
>
> Sentences that combine my experiences: Although I have made things happen in my life, I do not have the necessary support I need to get me through my treatments. I know I have had a strong will before to make these things happen, but I am feeling disillusioned.
>
> Sentences of support: It is true that I have been successful in the past, and it is also true that I will be successful now during my treatments, even without family support. I have wonderful friends who love me and who I can depend on to provide me all the emotional support I need. I can borrow from their strength.

Gateway 17

CLARITY

Clarity is the key to balance.

Look at the diagram on this page. Notice that it is in the shape of a scale. Copy this image in your journal and make a list, on the left side of the scale, of all the areas of your life that are in balance. Then, on the right side of the scale, make a list of all the things that are out of balance in your life. Be honest.

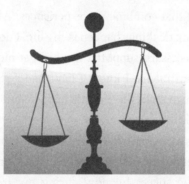

Take a look at your scale drawing and what you wrote, and notice which side is heavier. If you find that the scale is evenly weighted, congratulations! But don't be surprised or disappointed if your scale shows an imbalance. You can change it. Know that you can decide to take small steps to achieve balance in your life, steps that will lead you to greater clarity.

STEP 1: Write a list of all the areas in your life that are in need of balance. These are your "balance challenges." For example, your list might include:

- Feeling overwhelmed by household chores
- Being too tired to shop for groceries
- Needing to find a supportive person to drive you to the grocery store or to medical appointments
- Wanting to go to the park and walk every day but not feeling up to driving there
- Lacking the money to pay for treatments you would like to have

STEP 2: In this step, you will create "balance solutions." These solutions are not "what you wish would happen" — they are concrete solutions you can implement so you don't feel overwhelmed and so you can use your energy for self-healing. You can creatively solve challenges by enlisting the aid of others, and perhaps create solutions that you never would have previously considered. You may want to formulate your balance solutions with a close friend or family member who can share innovative ideas with you. Balance solutions can catapult you out of feeling victimized because they allow you to solve day-to-day problems and free yourself from the worry they can cause.

To create your balance solutions, take a sheet of paper and divide it into two columns. At the top of the left column, write the heading "Balance Challenge," and at the top of the right column, put the heading "Balance Solution." In the left column, list the balance challenges you identified in step 1. Then, in the right column, list possible solutions for each balance challenge. Here is an example:

BALANCE CHALLENGE	BALANCE SOLUTION
1. Overwhelmed by house-hold chores.	Hire a cleaning person to help you.
	Ask members of your family or friends (the people who ask what they can do to help) to commit to cleaning your house twice a week.
	Hire a trusted teenager in the neighborhood to help you.
	Contact your spiritual/religious community and let it be known you are looking for help.
2. Unable to shop for groceries because I'm too tired.	Ask family/friends for help and provide them with a shopping list.
	Order groceries online.
	Call up the manager of your local grocery store, and invite them to be part of your wellness plan. Ask them to set up an account so you can order online or by phone each week.

BALANCE CHALLENGE	BALANCE SOLUTION
3. Need to find someone I trust who can drive me to and from appointments when I'm not feeling well enough to drive.	Ask your healthcare professionals if they have any type of car service or patient advocate on staff who can help you.
	Contact local hospitals and ask to speak with an oncology social worker who may be able to give you suggestions.
	Contact your spiritual/religious community and let them know that you are seeking someone to help you.
	Ask family or friends to help you, and create a schedule for them.
	Take a cab.
	Call local oncology support communities and find out if they offer any type of transportation services.
	Contact the social work departments of local universities to find out if they have any health advocates who can help you arrange transportation.
	Find out about volunteer organizations in your community, including programs for recent retirees.

continued on the next page

BALANCE CHALLENGE	BALANCE SOLUTION
3. Need to find someone I trust who can drive me to and from appointments when I'm not feeling well enough to drive.	Call organizations in your community that offer support services for people with cancer and ask if they have anyone you can contact in your neighborhood. (In particular, sharing a drive to your appointments with someone who has navigated this journey can be very comforting.)
	Begin a "buddy system" program in your community that can help not only you, but other women who need assistance. You can also name the program after someone whose life has touched you.
	Contact the nursing programs at local schools for assistance; some of their students may be able to receive credit for advocacy and community involvement.

Using the balance solutions as a solid frame of reference can help you remove many of the perceived obstacles that have hindered you in the past. Don't be afraid to reach out and ask for help. Remember you are deserving of that help, so ask. You are not alone and not the only person who has felt overwhelmed, especially during treatments. Joan wasn't afraid to ask for help, and you can do the same. Perhaps you will be surprised and have the chance to meet new people and create meaningful friendships. It is not always easy to ask for help, and if you find you are having difficulty asking some-one, think about what a gift you are offering to that person — a chance to make a difference in your life by coming to your aid. That is an honorable feeling.

Gateway 18

❧❧❧

PERSONAL POWER

Retrieve your personal power.

When you retrieve your personal power, you are reminded of just how strong and mighty you truly are. Personal power is not power over others and does not involve any type of emotional manipulation. In order for you to retrieve your personal power and connect with what it feels like, it's helpful to begin with an excavation. This is an opportunity to truly examine (perhaps for the first time) what your beliefs are concerning personal power. Once you have observed how this power resides both inside and out and learned to retrieve and use this power, you will realize that your power is not just reserved for special times, but is an integral part of you.

STEP 1: I invite you to write a paragraph using the following sentence as your opening line. Begin by writing this sentence and let all of your thoughts about personal power unfold as you continue writing: "My personal power means _____."

STEP 2: Continue by completing this statement in one or more sentences: "I know when I give my power away because I feel _____."

STEP 3: Finish the exercise by completing this statement in one or more sentences: "The most recent experience I had of giving my power away occurred when _____."

STEP 4: This is the most important component of this exercise, and it is necessary to be completely honest so that the exercise has full value for you. If you need to set this exercise aside and come back to this step, that is fine. It is crucial that you only commit to what you truly believe. With those things in mind, write your thoughts by completing this statement with a description of steps you are willing to take: "I intend to reclaim my personal power. In order to do this, these are the steps I acknowledge I am willing to take at this time: _____."

Gateway 19

❧

PRIORITIZE

Give yourself permission to place yourself first.

Placing yourself first is now more important than ever. Most women possess a nurturing quality and fall into the trap of taking care of everyone else, all too often neglecting their own needs by placing themselves at the bottom — rock bottom — of the list. Sometimes this is necessary, but this is not one of those times. Denying your needs won't work, for they have a loud and insistent voice; they will continue to cry out for your attention until they are acknowledged and listened to. If you deny those voices, you will experience undue stress, exhaustion, frustration, and even rage. However, you can change that. In order to rectify the situation, you must first and foremost accept that you, my dear, are the priority. You come first. Period. This is the time, now, to make yourself the priority. This is not a selfish act. It provides you with validation that you can nurture yourself in the manner you deem appropriate.

STEP 1: Write your name on a blank sheet of paper in a beautiful color. Below your name, write all the actions that could support your psychological, spiritual, and physical self. What can you do right now that will serve your healing process?

List all activities that you can engage in that will truly serve you and aid in your wellness plan. For example, one woman's list included the following:

- Make time to call friends
- Make time to have lunch with friends
- Spend time in the park
- Have my nails done once a week
- Practice meditation
- Take a bath with scented candles
- Shut off the phone by 8 PM
- Read books I enjoy
- Take a day trip
- Practice yoga
- Attend a support group
- Paint
- Schedule a Reiki healing session
- Take myself out to breakfast each morning with a favorite person
- Go to the farmers' market

STEP 2: Now look at your list and cross off anything that you don't feel you have a strong connection with. Once you've finalized your list, take another look and choose a few activities from it that you can add to your schedule realistically. Put them on your schedule and commit to doing them. Honor this commitment.

Gateway 20

VICTORY SPONSOR

Find heroines in your life, real or imagined.

A victory sponsor is a mentor and companion during your healing journey who can offer you support, kindness, and compassion when you are in need. When you choose who will be a member of your victory sponsor team, select wisely. Include only people who have the ability to offer you support and guidance, and who know how to really listen and be present for you. Choose only people you trust and who you know would be pleased to be part of your healing team. You do not need a long list of people.

If you decide you would like to work with someone from history or literature, of course, you won't be able to connect with them in person, but that does not mean you can't create a connection. You can contact them through meditation, guided imagery, or imagined dialogue. Simply write your thoughts and feelings on a sheet of paper and ask for a response. The wealth of wisdom you receive through this dialogue may surprise you.

STEP 1: The key to this process is to identify your expectations and needs. Once you have a clear idea of what you need and what you expect of a victory sponsor, make a list of your victory sponsor requirements. Here is a sample list of expectations that reflects one woman's needs:

- My victory sponsor will call me twice a week to check in.
- My victory sponsor will be willing to be authentic and share her personal journey.
- My victory sponsor will be available to me to listen (and not talk) when I need them.
- My victory sponsor will be someone I can count on even during an emergency.

Feel free to adapt your list as your needs evolve over time.

STEP 2: Make a list of potential victory sponsors or select one person to be your victory sponsor. You may wish to choose a friend or family member, or other women who have traveled the cancer journey, to serve as your victory sponsor(s). Don't be afraid to ask your healing team if they can recommend someone who may be the perfect choice for your victory sponsor. Women's groups, cancer support organizations (both in your community and online), and counseling services may also prove helpful.

If you would rather work with a person from fiction or history as your victory sponsor, then take advantage of their courageous narrative as a source that you can rely on for inspiration. Visit your library or favorite bookstore, or call a cancer support organization and ask them if they have a list of inspirational books to recommend. Secondhand bookstores are wonderful places to discover a victory sponsor, and you may find someone (or something) that speaks to you in a book that was written decades or centuries ago.

You may wish to begin a victory sponsor program in your community to help others. If you've chosen a victory sponsor from history or literature, think about creating a victory sponsor group at a local hospital, support community, or healing center where women can discuss how their victory sponsors from history or literature have helped them.

Gateway 21

❧❧❧

GIFT OF TEARS

Allow yourself to feel.

Our bodies recognize the inherent wisdom of tears, and crying is a terrific release. Crying is an honorable act and permits all of your pent-up emotions to find a point of release if you permit it. All too often, crying is perceived as something negative, while in fact it can offer emotional liberation. When you allow yourself to cry in a safe place, you are able to let go of all the overwhelming feelings that you may be stuffing down inside yourself through withdrawal from others or through addictive behaviors. It takes a courageous woman to open up to her deep emotions. If you feel as if you are out of control and your heart's knowing tells you that you need help, seek professional support. Find your safe place to express these emotions with a trusted friend or experienced healer who is not afraid to witness your tears with you.

STEP 1: Complete the following sentences to truly explore your beliefs about expressing your emotions through tears:

I believe that if I cry in front of other people, I am

_____.

I believe that if I cry alone in the privacy of my home, then I am _____.

The last time I truly cried was when _____.

I am (or am not) willing to cry because _____.

STEP 2: When you are ready, spend some time reading over what you wrote in step 1. Examine how your beliefs are serving or sabotaging your emotional and spiritual terrain. Everyone is different; some women cry easily, while others never allow themselves to cry. Resist the impulse to judge yourself. If you find that crying is very challenging for you, rent a sad movie and allow yourself to cry. Remember that crying is an act of courage. The more you can permit the expulsion of your tears, whether you feel sad, angry, or frustrated, the more you will feel in control of your emotions rather than controlled by them. Be fearless! Crying is a profound act of emotional surrender and at this time may be the most therapeutic action you can take.

Gateway 22

❦

INVITE THE LIGHT

Allow the force of light to aid your healing journey.

Light healing has a distinguished history and is found in many cultures. Avicenna, the Persian physician and student of Aristotle, wrote in *The Canon of Medicine* about his use of color therapy with patients as a diagnostic tool. The ancient Egyptians documented cures using color remedies for specific diseases, and the *Nei Ching*, a Chinese medical text compiled over two thousand years ago that is also the foundation for acupuncture, records specific medical protocols ascertained by color diagnosis. The ancient Greek Asclepian dream temples were especially built to include natural-light remedies for the thousands of pilgrims seeking treatment. Today you will have the opportunity to experience light healing.

STEP 1: The color, or different frequencies, of light affects everyone differently. The use of light in meditation can be very powerful. Choose a color or colors that appeal to you; ignore the attributes usually associated with particular colors so you won't be swayed by them in your selection. Visit a paint store and ask for sample color swatches for the colors that attract you. You will be painting the walls of your inner home. When you are back home, cut out each color and place it in a large glass container. You will use these colors as an aid to meditation. Before meditating, close your eyes and ask what color your body needs right now for healing. Place your hand in the container and, with your eyes closed, retrieve a color. Then open your eyes and place the color in front of you. (Alternatively, you can choose healing stones of various colors, shapes, and textures, and place them in a glass bowl. Before meditating, you would select a stone to hold that will impart its healing properties to you. Before you work with stones, however, cleanse them in water and sea salt or place them outside to be cleansed by the light of the sun.)

STEP 2: When you are ready, look at the color you chose and write down any thoughts that come to mind or any immediate intuitive responses you have to this color. If it doesn't feel right, put it back in the container and choose another color the same way you did in step 1. Once you select a color that feels appropriate and has a spark for your energy field, write down all your thoughts about this color and how you intend to use it in your meditation. You can begin by writing a statement of intention to accompany your meditation. For example, "I chose the color blue to use in my meditation to heal my stress."

STEP 3: Draw the silhouette of your body and place it in front of you. Working with colored pens, or pastels, draw the colors that feel right to you at this time around your body, or in specific areas of your body that you would like to heal. A variation of this exercise is to draw the various rays of rainbow colors that appeal to you circling your body like a flume. When you are finished, place the drawing in front of you and, before your meditation, memorize the image so you can bring the colors directly inside your body or envelop your body in them. Experiment with what colors feel good to you to add to your vitality and peace of mind.

Gateway 23

━━◈━━

SECOND OPINIONS

It is wise.

It is *always* wise to have a second opinion from experts you trust to help you make decisions regarding your treatment options. You can choose to arrange consultations with recommended healers of various specialties, such as physicians, oncologists, surgeons, acupuncturists, herbalists, naturopaths, homeopaths, and energy healers. You are on a sacred mission for healing, so ask for referrals from those you trust. When you have the time and the inclination, conduct your own research to learn what the medical literature has published about a specific treatment protocol. Find out what your options may be. The more you are educated about all the possibilities, not just one or two options, the more confidence you will have to select the treatments that are best for you. Healing is not one-size-fits-all, and neither are you. You are unique.

STEP 1: Write a list of all your treatment options. Include the names and contact information of the practitioners or organizations that you can speak with for further education. Practitioners who charge exorbitant amounts of money or make unrealistic promises should be taken off your list immediately. While you are preparing this list, make sure to include information on any special out-of-pocket expenses (such as travel), waiting times, and the credentials of each person you might get a second or even third opinion from. Gather the facts, acquire wisdom, and empower yourself, because you are in charge of your own health decisions. This is a reminder that the members of your healthcare team work for you, and you can hire and fire them at will!

STEP 2: When you have met with all of the people you have chosen to meet, write a list of their names again. Say each name aloud and pay attention to your visceral response. How do you really feel about this member of your medical team? Is there a message for you? One woman told me that she continued to work with the same oncologist year after year because he was an excellent doctor — and I am sure that was true — but through the years of her chemotherapy, he refused to acknowledge her as he walked through the room, ignoring her completely. She was able to live with that, but it was apparent that his lack of compassion hurt her. Her physician certainly was an excellent clinician, but he had a long way to go to become an excellent human being.

Choose wisely. Select the healing team you deserve and select the qualities that are important to you. You can re-create your team as you continue to search, until you define the qualities you require and then find and select the important people you want to entrust with your precious life.

Gateway 24

⌘

INTEGRITY VOWS

Honor your promises.

We all have an internal compass, and we know deep inside when we are off course. The integrity vows that you create (and perhaps sometimes violate) remind you when you are not in sync with your highest purpose. In this exercise, you have the opportunity to craft your integrity vows and gain insight into the obstacles that prevent you from being in alignment with those vows.

STEP 1: Make a list of all the qualities you identify as important for writing your integrity vows, without editing yourself. For example: honesty; integrity; compassion for self and others; listening to your body. Examine your list carefully and cross off anything that does not truly serve you. When you are finished, complete this sentence in your journal: "My integrity vows include the qualities of _____." If you think it would be inspiring for you, carry your list of integrity vows with you as a reminder of your sacred contract with yourself.

STEP 2: This step is truly the most important, as long as you are honest with yourself. This part of the exercise is not easy to do. In one or more sentences, complete this statement: "I will know when I am not living my integrity vows when _____."

Gateway 25

~~~~~

MAKE SWEEPING CHANGES

Create a new healing vision for yourself.

Throughout your journey through life, you will make many changes as you evolve and experience your individual path. Change can be exhilarating, refreshing, and revitalizing, but it can also be scary and treacherous; it depends on your point of view. The upside of sweeping change is that you can't really predict how you will feel until the change occurs, and therein lies the rub. For those of us who want definite answers, the idea of stepping outside the box will not be easy to contemplate. However, if you reframe your thinking, you can embrace change as a vehicle for receiving new revelations about yourself. Can you take the plunge and step out of your comfort zone?

STEP 1: You will need the following items: magazines, photographs of yourself (from any age), a clear glass dish or plate, and a glue stick or glue gun. Place the magazines in front of you. Take your time and select images from the magazines that speak to you. Cut out any words from the magazines that feel empowering to you. Place the images in one pile and the words in another, and put the piles aside. Go through your magazine photographs and illustrations and select those that you have a kinship with and would like to work with. Set aside in another pile the personal photographs you have selected — these are the photographs of yourself. From the three piles, you will be creating a collage that depicts the change from the old you to the new you.

Place the glass dish in front of you and choose images that attract you from each pile; these should be the images that you would like to use to document your transformation. Resist the inclination to lay out all of the materials in a completed form; instead, let the process inform you. Begin by choosing a photograph, text, or image and placing it on the *back* of the dish so you can see the images you selected through the dish. Then repeat this process, adding photos, text, and images to your collage. Once you are content with your choices, use the glue stick or gun and place the glue on the front of the images, because you will be gluing those images on the back of the plate. It may seem odd to glue the front of the images, but this is the correct process. By placing the glue on the top of the images, you will be able to see them from underneath the plate or dish and they will be held securely.

As you design your dish or plate, you can cut the materials into shapes if you wish. Give yourself time to allow the images you are working with to slowly evolve into a new design. Creating this plate is very healing; it can also be very revealing because often the images you have selected contain their own narrative.

STEP 2: You can learn how the symbols on the glass speak to you by being mindful of their messages. What do you notice? In my experience, these collages often reflect what words cannot. Take your time to gaze deeply into the glass dish (or plate) and write down everything you see, intuit, and experience, without editing yourself. If you feel there is an overall message being communicated, don't doubt yourself — just write it down. The glass serves many purposes: not only is it a container to hold your images, but it is also fragile and transparent. Your collage can reveal the transparency of your life with authenticity, depicting both fragility and strength. Whenever you are ready, you can make new glass plates, creating a collection that illustrates your healing journey.

Gateway 26

❧❧❧

NOURISH YOURSELF

Choose nourishment that feeds your spirit.

Nourishment is beholden to the beholder and is not created equally. Everyone has different needs to nurture themselves. For some women, eating healthy food, sharing conversations with friends, reading spiritual or inspirational books, or walking in the park provides nourishment. The mind, the body, and the soul all demand nourishment, and it is important to identify and reclaim not only the types of nourishment you crave, but also the types you may need for optimum healing. This exercise will assist you in that quest.

STEP 1: Make a list for each of these categories: mind nourishment, body nourishment, and spirit nourishment. In each category, list everything you can think of that would provide nourishment. Ask yourself what would nourish your mind and heart. Do you want to have conversations? Read? Walk in nature? Ask yourself what would nourish your body. Are you eating poorly? Can you drink healthy smoothies, eat fruit and vegetables, or simply make better food choices to help your body heal?

Do you love yoga? Dance? Need a session of energetic

medicine? What would truly bring you spiritual nourishment? Do you need more quiet time alone? Time to attend spiritual or religious services? If you cannot attend those services, create a personal altar that reflects your spiritual journey and decorate it with sacred objects that nourish your soul.

STEP 2: When your list is complete, circle your priorities in each category and make a commitment to include these sources of nourishment in your life on a daily basis. You don't have to commit to everything on your list, but you can select a few of the things you've listed to begin your nourishment process. Nourishing yourself with food that provides sustenance and vitality is very important, of course; however, nourishing your psychological and spiritual self is just as important. Choose your sources wisely and according to your energy level.

Gateway 27

❦

SECRETS

Discover your sacred secrets for healing.

The secrets we hold close to us always contain truths, although sometimes those truths are not welcome. However, once revealed, these secrets can be our hidden treasure. Secrets are also of great value because they can serve to remind you that you know, deeply know, what you have survived. The protected spaces that you hold, when brought into consciousness, can be sacred teachers.

Secrets have an aura of magic to them, especially because they are private. They connote what is mysterious and often forbidden, which explains their allure. However, the emotional price of withholding secrets from yourself is sabotaging your peace of mind. It takes an enormous amount of energy to keep secrets from view. It is when we are willing to delve into the mystery of those secrets and allow them to surface that they can offer their magical release. That is the teaching.

Your secrets are a mirror to what you deem private and protected, and you are the only person who can decide how many of your secrets you wish to explore. Write down all of the secrets that you hold but have not been willing to unearth. Let all the secrets you have held deep within that are no longer necessary emerge. Can these secrets be used for your own healing journey? How?

STEP 1: In order to get started, write down and complete the following sentence and then see what else flows from your mind and pen:

The secrets I hold that I am willing to reveal are

_____.

STEP 2: Write a letter to yourself about the secrets you hold close and why you feel you must keep them private.

STEP 3: Write a letter to the person you would like to share your secrets with and explain why sharing these secrets will help you in your healing process. You can choose to mail the letter or not. If the letter is for someone who has passed away, write it to them and read it aloud. When you are finished, burn it.

~~~~⚮~~~~

ARMY OF SUPPORT

Create an army of support for yourself and your healing.

You do not have to be alone on your journey. You can have help; you deserve help. You will be creating the army of support that you need for your healing journey, an army that will sustain, nourish, and inspire you. Choose your army with discernment, for it will include important members of your healing team.

STEP 1: Create a list of all of the people you know that you can count on, truly count on.

STEP 2: Create a second list that reflects what your army of support would look like if you had all the assistance you need. Be honest and choose all the people you truly need. For example, your list might include:

- Someone to help you organize your appointments
- Someone to talk to when you are really scared
- A favorite animal to cuddle with (real or stuffed)
- Someone to cook for you

- Someone to help you find financial resources to pay for your treatments

Know that you will need to revamp the list that you are creating at this moment. Your army of support will change over time because your needs will change. Don't be afraid to ask for help from others, for it is necessary in order to create the beautiful army of support you are designing. Let your friends, coworkers, and family members know you are creating this army and would appreciate their assistance. There are countless organizations that support women during their cancer journeys, and it is worth your time and effort to find them. You may want to contact some of the organizations listed in the Resources section of this book. If a particular organization does not address your needs, ask them to recommend someone else you can contact. Just one resource or kind word may lead you to exactly what you are looking for, but you have to ask and make it known that you are looking to create your army.

Gateway 29

HEART REMEMBERING

Your heart holds great wisdom.

A pilgrim is traditionally defined as "one who travels to a shrine or a holy place as a religious act." This Gateway is asking you, "Where has your heart traveled? Where does your heart want to visit?" These questions provide insight for creating a sacred pilgrimage, real or imagined. You can travel to a place of great meaning for a heart pilgrimage. But you can also make that trip inside the sacred spaces of your home if you commit to spending time in silence, shutting off any distractions, in order to honor your heart pilgrimage.

It is not unusual for past hurts and wrongs to resurface when we are feeling vulnerable. This exercise provides you with protection for exploring those areas so you can create a new way of understanding and work with the energies of what your heart remembers.

STEP 1: Answer the following questions by writing down what comes to mind immediately, without editing yourself:

What does your heart remember?
Who has your heart not forgiven?

If you left the world tomorrow, would your heart
have any regrets?

Where does your heart wish to travel?

STEP 2: When you are finished, reflect on your answers to gain further insights. This is an introspective process and may take many days, even weeks, to complete. So don't be discouraged if it takes you a long time.

Gateway 30

YOU ARE A HEROINE

You are a heroine in your own journey.

This is a potent writing exercise and offers you an opportunity to place yourself in a narrative as the main character. It is an exercise to remind you that you are the heroine that you seek.

STEP 1: Write your story, beginning with what you remember from the time when you first received your diagnosis and continuing up to where you are now. Make sure you include the courage you have exhibited and the strength you possess, for those qualities, although challenged at times, will not be diminished. You can even choose a new name for yourself that reflects the heroine that you are.

STEP 2: When you have time, rent the film *Joan of Arc* with Ingrid Bergman, for inspiration (there are many films on Joan of Arc, but this is my favorite). If that is not enough, find a heroine in mythology, or in art or literature, to inspire you. When you are finished writing the story of your journey, read it aloud. You may choose to share your unique story with others, for it is a story of courage and inspiration that can help others on a similar path.

CREATE YOUR OWN MANTRA

Choose the message you need to receive.

This Gateway is yours to invent. Take your time and think about a message you would like to hear, one that would make all the difference to you. Make a list of everything you wish people would say to you but don't. You can also choose to write a list of messages that come directly from your soul self. The only criterion is to make sure that whatever you write contains messages of support that you need in your life right now.

When you are finished writing your messages, choose one that calls to you and speaks your truth directly, and place this message in front of you. Study the message and when you are ready, write, in a stream-of-consciousness fashion, whatever comes to mind when you reflect on the message you have chosen. Let the pen guide you and don't worry about grammar, spelling, or punctuation.

Put the rest of your messages on small slips of paper. Each day, in the morning or before you start your daily routine, choose one message. You may wish to tuck a message into your pocket or carry one with you when you go to treatment or a medical appointment. You can also hold it in your mind and simply reflect on its message.

Afterword

LIVING YOUR FLAME OF COURAGE

Healing is a personal and sacred journey, and is unique for everyone. Your healing journey will not look or feel like anyone else's, but healing in its myriad forms is always available to you. I remember that my shamanic teacher often reminded me that healing has many shapes and not to judge the package it arrives in. The root of the word *heal* is the Old English word *haelan*, which is related to the idea of becoming whole. Noted psychotherapist and physician Carl Jung created the concept of individuation, a lifelong process of becoming whole — a process that is centered around one's individuality and innermost uniqueness.

I propose that the journey of illness can activate your spiritual journey and become your soul's journey as you, like Joan of Arc, discover what your special gifts and purpose are. The challenges of a cancer diagnosis offer you the opportunity to reveal what is most important to you during your soul journey. It is not unusual to feel that this diagnosis is a personal failure and to be unsure of what decisions to make next. This helplessness can be altered by learning to listen to your body's wisdom, building strong support systems, and creating a milieu of trust with your healthcare providers.

You may be transformed physically and emotionally

by pharmaceutical therapies, chemotherapy, surgery, radiation, catheterization, port insertions, biopsies, and other invasive procedures. These physical changes are powerful; they will alter your psyche and spirit, and are not to be diminished. Joan's flame of courage burned brightly as her old self underwent a metamorphosis to make way for her new self. That was and is the core of her journey and yours. I hope the guidance in this book has helped you understand that your vulnerability and nakedness of both body and soul can be the catalyst for lasting transformation, beauty, and empowerment.

The word for "understanding" in the Thai language translates to "entering the heart." You can teach your healthcare team that their gifts of attention and presence are not only compassionate acts, but also medicinal and needed. Joan of Arc recognized that sanctity by honoring her gift of attention and the presence of her voices, her true companions throughout her life. She wasn't afraid to express her soul's directives even in the most challenging of times.

I appreciate the philosophy of William Osler, who is often considered the father of contemporary medicine, just as Asclepius (whose caduceus is the insignia of the medical profession) and Hippocrates were considered the fathers of ancient medicine. Osler elegantly lectured to medical students, stating that healing occurs when physicians learn to view patients *as people and not as their disease*: "The good physician treats the disease; the great physician treats the patient who has the disease." He was speaking about addressing the mind, body, and spirit.

When anyone receives a life-changing diagnosis, compassion is not only foundational, but an ethical consideration and just as important as treating the disease. Evidence of that caring connection is demonstrated by a physician-healer who explains a treatment plan in detail to alleviate your panic; a physician-healer who returns a phone call while you are awaiting serious test results; or a physician-healer who takes the time to visit you in the hospital just to see how you are doing or drops by during treatments to offer a friendly smile and reassurance. In fact, I believe that without compassion, one isn't truly practicing medicine. Excellence in clinical care is a requirement, but excellence in compassionate care that includes all parts of you should also be part of the equation. This is your right, and if you don't receive it, keep looking for professionals who can provide you with the full spectrum of healing.

You can activate your flame of courage and make a significant impact on the medical culture by speaking up and insisting that you receive excellence in clinical as well as compassionate care. Allow yourself to guide your caregivers and practitioners toward compassionate medicine. I would like to offer you a code of healing that you can easily adopt to guide you to further healing of heart, mind, and body. If Joan of Arc had cancer, she would endorse this code, for it reflects the courage, honor, and integrity that she possessed, as you do.

CODE OF HEALING

I have built an army of support of loving and healing people in my life.

I have chosen a healing team of practitioners who reflect wisdom, compassion, and excellence in their clinical skills.

I expect to receive support, caring, and compassionate medicine from all members of my healthcare team.

I insist that all of my healthcare providers answer all of my (and my loved ones') questions about any medical procedure, medication, or treatment until I am satisfied with the answers so that I understand fully before making decisions about my care.

I will seek out practitioners who can educate me about treatment options and who will make sure that I know what I can expect from each option.

I expect my healthcare providers to return my calls in a timely manner.

I will share my spiritual and religious preferences with my healthcare team.

I will only ask for help from people in my army of support who can honor my requests.

I am willing to create boundaries for myself. When I am not feeling well, I will not push myself, and I will listen to my body's wisdom.

I will seek out spiritual support from my community when I need it.

I honor kindness, for myself and others.

I will not be stingy with myself or hold back from insisting that I deserve the best, not only in my cancer journey, but in all areas of my life. I will not wait for the "right time" to do this.

I am willing to be a "teacher" to my physician and share my wisdom.

I honor my journey every step of the way.

Joan of Arc demonstrated during her trial that she was a woman of power, conviction, and nobility, and she continues to serve as a sage hundreds of years after her death. I hope that, in working with this book, you have been surprised by what you have learned about yourself and have realized that the flame of courage you possess is just as noble as Joan of Arc's, because that is true. I also hope that Joan's unwavering courage in the face of great adversity has provided inspiration for you to seize your personal power as she did, to create a life that honors you. I invite you to enjoy the meditations in the Flames of Courage section of the book again and again, because I believe they will help you attain the quiet to listen to your own healing voice, as Joan so artfully did in her own life.

In Native American culture, medicine means more than a substance to restore health and vitality to an ill body. Medicine means power, a vital energy that can be retrieved and directed for healing. Medicine also means knowledge. Trust yourself to delve deeper into your knowledge and power during the healing journey, now and for the rest of your life. I truly hope that you have discovered and embodied the rich and deep understanding of the wisdom of your flame of courage, which will live inside of you during both the good and the challenging times of your life, with Joan of Arc at your side. May it be so.

ACKNOWLEDGMENTS

This book is, and will always be, for my mother, whose heart of courage will continue to inspire me throughout my life. For Sidney, my dad and knight in shining armor, whose cancer journey was valiantly fought. I miss you both.

I want to acknowledge all of the women I have worked with over the years who have shared their soulful journeys with me. And to Jane Grossenbacher, your laughter is remembered.

I recognize just how fortuitous it was for me to be intuitively guided to the amazing Rita Rosenkranz. Thank you, Rita, for your unwavering support, literary acumen, and, most important, for continuing to believe in this project when others did not.

Georgia Hughes, you have brought kindness and an elegant commitment to this book, and working with you has been such a blessing. Thank you so much for bringing this book into form.

NOTES

Unless otherwise indicated, all quotes in this book are excerpts from the trial of Joan of Arc. These excerpts are based on the Orléans manuscript, which is considered the most accurate source, and are taken from the standard English translation of that manuscript, *The Trial of Joan of Arc: Being the Verbatim Report of the Proceedings from the Orleans Manuscript*, trans. W. S. Scott (London: Folio Society, 1956).

Introduction

Page 10 *records indicate that Joan slept*: Régine Pernoud and Marie-Véronique Clin, *Joan of Arc: Her Story*, ed. Bonnie Wheeler, trans. Jeremy duQuesnay Adams (New York: St. Martin's Press, 1999), 104.

Page 12 *"Certain enemies betrayed her"*: Ibid., 157.

Page 12 *"Search as you may"*: Sieur Louis de Conte [Mark Twain], "Personal Recollections of Joan of Arc," *Harper's Magazine*, 1896.

Page 16 *"the simplicity of wabi sabi"*: Leonard Koren, *Wabi-Sabi for Artists, Designers, Poets & Philosophers* (Point Reyes, CA: Imperfect Publishers, 2008), 72.

Page 16 *"Pare down the essence"*: Ibid.

Flame of Courage 6: Trust

Page 45 *"When she was watching"*: Pernoud and Clin, *Joan of Arc*, 28.

Flame of Courage 17: Clarity

Page 71   *Jamie Sams describes the voice*: Jamie Sams, *Dancing the Dream: The Seven Sacred Paths of Human Transformation* (New York: HarperOne, 1999), 175.

Flame of Courage 21: Gift of Tears

Page 84   *"Joan has great distinction"*: Léon Cristiani, *St. Joan of Arc: Virgin-Soldier* (Boston: St. Paul Editions, 1977), 82.

Flame of Courage 22: Invite the Light

Page 85   *"ring the bells"*: Leonard Cohen, "Anthem," from *Stranger Music: Selected Poems and Songs* (New York: Random House, 1994), 373.

Flame of Courage 25: Make Sweeping Changes

Page 97   *"one of the guards wished"*: Pernoud and Clin, *Joan of Arc*, 105.

Flame of Courage 30: You Are a Heroine

Page 111   *"Surrender to the Maid"*: Pernoud and Clin, *Joan of Arc*, 34.

Gateway 3: Surrender

Page 128   *"sage is like a person"*: Kenneth Cohen, *Honoring the Medicine: The Essential Guide to Native American Healing* (New York: Ballantine Books, 2006), 128. This book is one of my favorites, and he explains the use of sage in ceremony in detail.

Afterword: Living Your Flame of Courage

Page 200   *"The good physician treats"*: Robert M. Centor, MD, "To Be a Great Physician, You Must Understand the Whole Story," *Medscape General Medicine* 9(1): 59, published online March 26, 2007, www.ncbi.nlm.hih.gov/pmc/articles/PMC1924990.

RESOURCES

The following are organizations and practitioners devoted to helping people with cancer.

Organizations and Educational Resources

1 IN 8 FOUNDATION
Dedicated to addressing early cancer detection and awareness.
www.1in8.org

AMERICAN ASSOCIATION FOR CANCER RESEARCH
Offers a wealth of information on support groups and a database of organizations that provide cancer-related services.
615 Chestnut St., 17th Floor
Philadelphia, PA 19106
866-423-3965
aacr@aacr.org
www.aacr.org

THE ANNIE APPLESEED PROJECT
Provides information, education, and advocacy for people with cancer, their family and friends. Sponsors an annual evidence-based complementary and alternative cancer therapies conference.
7319 Serrano Ter.
Delray Beach, FL 33446
561-749-0084
annieappleseedpr@aol.com
www.annieappleseedproject.org

BEYOND BOOBS! INC.

Not your typical support group, Beyond Boobs! offers encouragement, support, and education on breast cancer.

1311 Jamestown Rd., #202
Williamsburg, VA 23185
757-645-2649
checkthemout@beyondboobs.org
www.beyondboobs.org

BRIDGE FOR HEALING CANCER and BRIDGE FOR HEALING CANCER PODCASTS

Nicki Scully, Alchemical Healing Practitioner
Phone bridge rituals conducted by Nicki Scully to heal and transform cancer.

www.shamanicjourneys.com/cancerbridge.php
www.planetaryhealingbook.com

CANCER SUPPORT COMMUNITY

Home to affiliated support communities: Gilda's Club Worldwide, The Wellness Community

888-793-9355 (helpline)
www.cancersupportcommunity.org

CURE MAGAZINE

Free online magazine combining science with humanity for people with cancer.

www.curetoday.com

FROM CHRYSALIS TO WINGS PSYCHOTHERAPY AND RESEARCH CENTER

Home of A Way of Life after Breast Cancer; offers retreats for breast cancer survivors.

949-916-6851
francine@chrysalistowings.com
www.chrysalistowings.com

Healing Journeys

An organization whose mission statement is to support healing, activate hope, and promote thriving; offers free Cancer as a Turning Point™ conference.

> PO Box 221417
> Sacramento, CA 95822
> 800-423-9882
> info@healingjourneys.org
> www.healingjourneys.org

Pink-Link

Connecting breast cancer survivors since 2006; Vicki Tashman, founder.

> 310-995-5204
> www.pink-link.org
> www.cansurvivorblog.com

Sharsheret

National nonprofit organization supporting young women and their families, of all Jewish backgrounds, facing breast cancer.

> 866-474-2774
> info@sharsheret.org
> www.sharsheret.org

Stand Up to Cancer

A program of the Entertainment Industry Foundation, whose mission is to raise funds for research. Website lists a variety of advocacy, support, and cancer research resources.

> www.standup2cancer.org

Financial Aid

My Hope Chest

Funds reconstruction surgery for breast cancer survivors.

> 727-488-0320
> info@myhopechest.org
> kimberly.hall@myhopechest.org
> www.myhopechest.org

PATIENT ADVOCATE FOUNDATION

Helps patients solve insurance and healthcare access problems.

> 800-532-5274
> help@patientadvocate.org
> www.patientadvocate.org

THE PINK FUND

Provides up to ninety days of nonmedical financial aid to cover basic costs of living.

> 877-234-7465
> www.thepinkfund.org

THE CATHERINE H. TUCK FOUNDATION

Provides financial aid for women with breast cancer.

> 1507 7th St., #602
> Santa Monica, CA 90401
> info@catherinefund.org
> www.catherinefund.org

Practitioners

ROSEMARY BOURNE

Acupuncture.

> PO Box 2427
> Telluride, CO 81435
> 415-461-6641
> rosemary@colorpuncture.com
> www.colorpunctureusa.com

ELIZABETH CARR, ACUPUNCTURE PHYSICIAN

Oncology support.

> 925 5th Ave. Pkwy.
> Naples, FL 34102
> 239-860-8660
> beth@bethcarr.com
> www.bethcarr.com

CENTER FOR HEALTH & HUMAN DEVELOPMENT
Kenneth Zeno, MA, MAT, ABD (PhD)
Healthy lifestyles specialist; Duke University–certified integrative health coach.

> 561-654-9449
> ken@healthcoachzeno.com
> www.healthcoachzeno.com

CLEARING CLOUDS ENERGETIC MEDICINE
Sessions by phone or Skype. Clearing Clouds is a somatic, intuitive process that addresses the root cause of physical and emotional pain.

> Jyoti SaeUn
> Oakland, CA
> 510-923-9057
> clearingclouds@gmail.com
> www.clearingclouds.com

VICKI NOBLE
Feminist healer offering soul-based, intuitive astrology readings.

> www.motherpeace.com

NUTRITIONAL SOLUTIONS
Nutritional oncology.
Jeanne M. Wallace, PhD, CNC

> 1697 E. 3450 North
> North Logan, UT 84341
> 435-563-0053
> www.nutritional-solutions.net

PROVIDENCE WHOLISTIC HEALTHCARE
Integrative oncology support.

> Sheila M. Frodermann, MA, ND, FHANP
> Carol L. Seng, MAOM, LAc
> 144 Waterman St., #3
> Providence, RI 02906
> 401-455-0546
> providencewholistic@gmail.com
> www.providencewholistic.com

THE RED TENT
Healing arts for women.
> Lisa Kelly, LMT
> 4838 NW 2nd Ave.
> Boca Raton, FL 33431
> 561-865-5791
> direct: 954-295-3870
> lisa@redtentwellness.com
> www.redtentwellness.com

JUDITH THOMPSON, ND
Customized holistic wellness for women.
> 503-314-9858
> DrJudithND@aol.com

HELAYNE WALDMAN, MS, EdD, CNE
Holistic nutrition practitioner and coauthor of *The Whole-Food Guide for Breast Cancer Survivors*.
> www.turning-the-tables.com
> www.wholefoodguideforbreastcancer.com

ABOUT THE AUTHOR

Janet Lynn Roseman, PhD, is an assistant professor in medical education at Nova Southeastern University College of Osteopathic Medicine in Fort Lauderdale, Florida, and director of the Physician Fellowship Program in Integrative Medicine. She specializes in spirituality and medicine, and created the Sidney Project in Spirituality and Medicine and Compassionate Care™, a unique model in medical education that reminds physician residents of the sacredness of their profession and the importance of creating caring environments for both patients and physicians. She was the David Larsen Fellow in Spirituality and Medicine at the Kluge Center for Scholars at the Library of Congress.

She leads workshops for people with cancer and offers the "Cultivating Courage with Joan of Arc" training program for healthcare professionals who work with oncology patients. She lectures on the intersection of compassion and medicine, and is dedicated to changing the medical culture from what it is to what it can be. Dr. Roseman is also a Reiki master, dance therapist, and intuitive healer and has worked with oncology patients using color and light therapy. Her column on healing with Joan of Arc often appears in *Sedona Journal of Emergence*. She can be contacted at dancejan@aol.com.

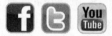